D0338794

DISCARD

THE HEALTHY SKEPTIC

DISCARD

THE HEALTHY SKEPTIC

CUTTING THROUGH THE HYPE ABOUT YOUR HEALTH

ROBERT J. DAVIS, PHD

UNIVERSITY OF CALIFORNIA PRESS

BERKELEY   LOS ANGELES   LONDON

DISCARD

University of California Press, one of the most distinguished university presses in the United States, enriches lives around the world by advancing scholarship in the humanities, social sciences, and natural sciences. Its activities are supported by the UC Press Foundation and by philanthropic contributions from individuals and institutions. For more information, visit www.ucpress.edu.

University of California Press
Berkeley and Los Angeles, California

University of California Press, Ltd.
London, England

© 2008 by Robert J. Davis

Library of Congress Cataloging-in-Publication Data

Davis, Robert J., 1963–
    The healthy skeptic : cutting through the hype about your health / Robert J. Davis.
        p.   cm.
    Includes bibliographical references and index.
    ISBN 978-0-520-24918-9 (cloth : alk. paper)
    1. Health education.   2. Consumer education.   3. Health products. 4. Quacks and quackery.   5. Health—Information services.   I. Title.
RA440.5.D38   2008
613—dc22   2007037341

Manufactured in the United States of America

17   16   15   14   13   12   11   10   09   08
10 9 8 7 6 5 4 3 2 1

This book is printed on Natures Book, which contains 50% post-consumer waste and meets the minimum requirements of ANSI/NISO z39.48-1992 (R 1997) (*Permanence of Paper*).

FOR MY MOTHER
AND
IN MEMORY OF MY FATHER

CONTENTS

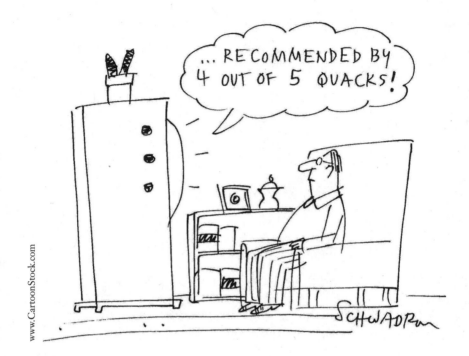
www.CartoonStock.com

INTRODUCTION
HEALTH SELLERS

N early all of us can point to particular moments, often seemingly inconsequential at the time, that ended up affecting our lives in profound and lasting ways. For me, such an instant came during my sophomore year of college and involved, of all things, milk. When the topic somehow came up at lunch one day, I bragged to friends that my highly enlightened family had always shunned whole milk and restricted ourselves to 2 percent, the type that's low in fat. Basking in my own virtuousness, I couldn't stop there. As they downed their glasses of whole milk, I advised my friends that they would be smart to follow my example and switch to 2 percent.

Overhearing all this was a know-it-all kid from New Jersey named Marty. "Actually," he said, inserting himself into our conversation, "2 percent milk is not really low in fat."

"Yes, it is," I shot back. "It says so on the carton."

Armed for battle, Marty didn't miss a beat: "Well, the carton lies. The fat content in 2 percent is closer to whole milk than to skim milk. If you want low fat, you need to drink skim or 1 percent."

My friends watched in silence. Now it was my turn. Unable to present any facts to refute Marty's argument, all I could come up with was, "I think you're wrong."

That afternoon, I headed to the library in search of the truth. (Believe it or not, young readers, there once was no Internet, nor were foods required to have nutrition labels.) Poring over the dusty pages of a nutrition textbook, I discovered, much to my chagrin, that a glass of 2 percent milk has about 5 grams of fat, compared to 8 grams in whole milk and nearly 0 in skim. Know-it-all Marty, it turned out, knew exactly what he was talking about.

How was it, I wondered, that Marty was so well informed, while I, the son of a doctor (as if this had any relevance), had been in the dark? What else did I not know about diet and health? I started to read everything I could get my hands on. The more I learned, the more intrigued I became—and the more I came to question what I thought I knew. In time, my newfound interest in health would become a passion, both personally and professionally.

That quest to get to the truth, born of my humbling exchange with Marty, continues to this day. It's what motivates me as a health and medical journalist. And it's the driving force behind this book.

Everywhere we turn, it seems, we're bombarded with information about how to stay healthy: Have some green tea. Take an aspirin. Eat soy. Cut out carbs. Avoid plastic bottles. Take antioxidants. Use hormones. Don't use hair dye. Get tested. Meditate. The list goes on and on.

If there's one complaint I hear more than any other from viewers and readers, it's that they're overwhelmed and uncertain about what advice to believe. One woman summed it up this way: "I consider myself above average in paying attention to items concerning health. . . . But there is such a glut of junk information, it is really difficult to sort out the good from the bad."

It would be nearly impossible to write a book sorting through every single claim about health and wellness. There are simply too many, and new ones emerge every day. But it is possible to equip you to become your own health information detective, so that you can identify the motives and "weapons" of those who are disseminating advice and verify whether there's adequate evidence to back up their claims. With a better understanding of who's behind the information and where to go to check it out, you'll be in a stronger position to determine what's believable and what's not. That's what being a healthy skeptic is all about.

SELLING HEALTH

Certainly, the practice of urging people to lead healthier lives is nothing new. In 1928, a prominent public health official named Dr. Herman Bundesen called for a new approach to health promotion. (Though that term can have different meanings, I use it in this book to refer to efforts to educate and encourage the public to adopt healthful practices. I call those behind such efforts "health promoters.") Bundesen, recognizing the ascendancy of mass media, advertising, and marketing in American culture, urged that they be harnessed to improve public health. In a speech titled "Selling Health—A Vital Duty," he said to his colleagues: "My plea is that you live health, talk health, sell health, and think health. Sell it alike to young and old. Sell it by example and precept; by good health news published in the right way; through the press; by the motion picture, the radio, slogan and poster, or in any other way you will. But *sell* it."

Today, the "selling" of health has far surpassed anything Bundesen likely ever imagined. Television, radio, newspapers, magazines, books, newsletters, and the Internet inundate us with the latest ways to be healthier and live longer. Companies blast us with ubiquitous advertising for foods, beverages, drugs, vitamins, herbs, and other products that promise to keep us healthy. Doctors and diet gurus preach the virtues of their particular wellness and weight loss regimens through books, media appearances, and lectures. Spas, fitness facilities, and "longevity" clinics promote regimens intended to boost our health. Celebrities on health crusades advise us, as do consumer activists and health groups. Government health agencies issue a steady stream of alerts, advisories, pamphlets, and public service announcements, all intended to prevent disease and promote wellness. Even the relatively staid Centers for Disease Control and Prevention (CDC) has an entire center devoted to what it calls "health marketing."

Fueling this explosion of selling is our seemingly insatiable demand for ways to stay healthy. Baby boomers, not content to passively accept illness, disability, and death as their forebears often did, have led the way in trying to head off, or at least delay, the inevitable.

Our changing health care system has also helped stoke demand. Previously, people got information about health and wellness mainly from their doctors. But now, with only a few minutes allotted to see each patient, most doctors have little time to discuss matters like diet, exercise, or environmental hazards. And in many cases, physicians aren't especially knowledgeable about such subjects; their training generally involves how to fix problems, not prevent them. As a result, people have increasingly turned elsewhere for guidance.

Advances in the science of wellness have played a role, too. With prevention-related research receiving greater visibility, prestige, and funding during the past few decades, we've seen an explosion of knowledge about the possible causes of various conditions and the best ways to reduce our risk. And more knowledge means there's more than ever to sell.

There are also more opportunities to sell, thanks to the rapid proliferation in recent years of consumer publications, cable channels, and, of course, the Internet, which has given health selling the unprecedented reach and power it has today. One wonders what Dr. Bundesen would make of it all.

THE HEALTH PROMOTION "INDUSTRY"

It's no secret that many of those engaged in selling health are out to make a buck. Or big bucks. Economist Paul Zane Pilzer estimates that the wellness industry will be worth $1 trillion by 2010, as baby boomers spend more and more on products and services that promise to promote longer and healthier lives. In a book instructing readers "how to make a fortune in the next trillion dollar industry," Pilzer writes that "a few wellness entrepreneurs . . . will emerge as the billionaires and media darlings of our new century. Hundreds of thousands more . . . will become millionaires."

For other health sellers, the driving force isn't money but attention. By promoting a particular cause, they can burnish their reputations and enhance their careers; or, if they lead an advocacy group, they can boost its visibility. Others simply want to improve public health. Perhaps they're driven by evangelistic zeal, resembling Bundesen in viewing the selling of their particular cause as a "vital duty." For still others, there's a combination of altruism and self-interest at work.

Given their varying motives, disparate sellers such as product marketers, diet book authors, consumer activists, and government health officials probably don't think of themselves as having much in common. Some would even take umbrage at being lumped together with others whom they consider far less ethical or high-minded. But the fact is that regardless of what drives them, all are involved in basically the same pursuit: trying to influence what we know, believe, and do when it comes to our health. For consumers, who are constantly bombarded with health-related advice from all directions, the messages are often indistinguishable. In essence, these sellers are all part of a massive health promotion "industry." And, yes, as a health journalist—and the author of this book—I am certainly a member of it.

Sellers in this industry have to compete for consumers' attention in a crowded and competitive marketplace of goods and ideas, where it's usually necessary to have a loud voice and bold claims to be heard. Whether the message is in the form of a news report, an ad, or a slogan for an awareness-raising campaign, sellers strive to make it simple and unambiguous, lest consumers tune it out and focus their attention elsewhere. To convey complex scientific information in this environment, health promoters may resort to oversimplifying or sensationalizing. They may not necessarily lie to us, but, like anyone else trying to sell something, they don't always tell us the full truth, either. Instead, what we may get, even from individuals and organizations with the most altruistic of motives, is hype, half-truths, and spin.

Sometimes, it's perfectly obvious we're being spun: think TV infomercials for ab-flattening exercise machines or Internet ads for waist-shrinking herbal supplements. Generally, we recognize sales efforts like these for what they are—propaganda by manufacturers to entice us to buy products—and we know not to take them as gospel. But in many more cases, it's not so clear what health promoters' agendas might be or how they might be stretching the truth in order to influence us. In fact, some sellers are invisible, working behind the scenes to sway us so that we are not even aware of it.

HORMONE THERAPY HYPE

The selling of hormone replacement therapy serves as a classic example—and a cautionary tale—of how the health promotion industry can lead us astray. The story begins with Dr. Robert Wilson, a gynecologist whose 1966 best-selling book, *Feminine Forever*, called menopause a "staggering catastrophe" that turns a woman into a "castrate," a "shrunken hag," and a "dull-minded but sharp-tongued caricature of her former self." Replacing lost estrogen, he said, could head off these horrors and keep women youthful-looking and "adaptable, even-tempered, and generally easy to live with." An excerpt from Wilson's book in *Look* magazine helped add to the buzz, as did articles in women's magazines that included statements such as this: "There doesn't seem to be a sexy thing estrogen can't and won't do to keep you flirtatiously feminine." Thanks to such hype, sales of the leading estrogen replacement drug, Premarin, skyrocketed. Unbeknownst to the public, though, Wilson's book and his foundation, which promoted hormone therapy, were funded by Premarin's manufacturer, Wyeth-Ayerst.

The drug's popularity temporarily waned in the 1970s after reports that it increased cancer of the lining of the uterus. But its reputation was rehabilitated when doctors determined that this problem could be addressed by combining estrogen with another hormone, progestin. Sales climbed again in the 1980s when hormone replacement therapy (HRT) was promoted for a new use: preventing the bone-loss disease osteoporosis. An awareness-raising campaign, funded by Wyeth, warned women about the devastating effects of bone loss and advised them to see their doctors.

Meanwhile, some research was suggesting that hormones might also prevent heart disease. Though the studies revealed only an association, not cause and effect, the news media often mischaracterized the evidence as a slam dunk. As Barbara Seaman wrote in her book *The Greatest Experiment Ever Performed on Women:* "The press, whether through intentional, drug-dollar-fueled deceit or simple negligence or oversight, continued for years to advocate as virtual fact a connection between heart and hormone."

As preliminary evidence emerged that HRT might also prevent other conditions, ranging from arthritis to Alzheimer's disease, media reports breathlessly played up these benefits while giving short shrift to possible risks, including breast cancer and blood clots. An article in *Newsweek* went so far as to exclaim that "years of research have painted [HRT] as the closest science has ever come to putting youth in a little oval tablet."

Enthusiastic pronouncements like these were encouraged by a steady stream of press releases and other materials from public relations firms that manufacturers had hired to promote HRT's benefits. Prominent experts who were unabashed cheerleaders for HRT added to the frenzy. For example, one well-known obstetrician-gynecologist, appearing on NBC's *Today*

Show, gushed that "if there was a similar medication that could do the same for men that [HRT] does for women, it would be in the cabinets in the bathrooms of every home in America."

Other doctors expressed their irrational exuberance through books with titles such as *Estrogen: How and Why It Can Save Your Life*. In one such book, the authors could barely contain their excitement in describing hormone therapy as a virtually risk-free preventive panacea:

> It is safe today. In fact, it is *better* than safe. . . . It will cut your risk of heart disease in half and prevent osteoporosis, the brittle bones disease. All indications are that it delays or prevents the development of Alzheimer's disease and improves age-related memory loss. It can prevent macular degeneration, an eye condition that can cause blindness, and the onset of cataracts. Most important, according to the foremost experts in the field, it will NOT put you at higher risk of developing breast cancer.

What the public typically didn't know was that this book's co-author, Dr. Lila Nachtigall, and some other frequently quoted HRT experts were the recipients of speaking fees, research grants, or other funding from pharmaceutical companies, including Wyeth. The drug maker also paid celebrities such as Lauren Hutton to sing the praises of hormone replacement. In a story in *Parade* magazine, the former supermodel (who was featured on the cover) called estrogen "my No. 1 secret" and proclaimed that "if I had to choose between all my creams and makeup for feeling and looking good, I'd take the estrogen."

But not everyone was jumping on the bandwagon. Some doctors and health groups expressed skepticism, pointing out that while HRT's ability to control menopausal symptoms and prevent thinning bones was well established, many of the other purported benefits were not. And it wasn't clear, they warned, that the risks were as minimal as many assumed.

Though their voices were generally drowned out by those of HRT enthusiasts, the skeptics were eventually vindicated by a landmark federal study known as the Women's Health Initiative. In 2002, the government announced it was halting the huge randomized clinical trial (the most definitive type of study, capable of showing cause and effect) because HRT was doing more harm than good. Women taking combination hormone therapy were less likely to have hip fractures and colon cancer than those on placebos—but they also had a small increase in their risk of heart attacks, strokes, and breast cancer. Later findings would show that they were also *more* prone to develop dementia.

Still, this was just one study (albeit the largest and most definitive to date) and involved just one type of HRT. Contrary to what some concluded, it did not prove that HRT was worthless or harmful for all women. But it did poke a huge hole in the HRT enthusiasts' case that most postmenopausal women should take hormones because the benefits far outweighed the risks.

The news that HRT was not all it had been cracked up to be came as a bombshell to many women, who felt confused and betrayed. They wondered how the advice they had heard for so long from so many people could have been so wrong. The answer, according to best-selling author Dr. Susan Love, was that "we made observations and developed hypotheses—and then forgot to prove them." Or, as women's health advocate Cynthia Pearson put it, the belief that hormones could prevent disease was "a triumph of marketing over science."

THE WHOLE TRUTH?

This kind of misleading health selling, often from sources we trust, isn't unique to HRT. We encounter it every day regarding all kinds of issues. Consider, for example, these statements:

Eating walnuts or chocolate can help ward off disease.

Going on a diet will make you healthier.

Early detection saves lives.

Sunscreen prevents skin cancer.

High cholesterol is a killer.

Taking vitamins is beneficial.

Commonly used products contain harmful chemicals.

We hear such pronouncements so often that few of us think to question them. But, in fact, they're not really facts. They're half-truths—oversimplified assertions with a kernel of truth, some that are based on less than definitive evidence and others that don't apply in all cases. Yet all are being peddled as absolute truths by various sellers in the health promotion industry.

In the chapters that follow, I dissect these notions and others like them, showing how they're misleading and who's behind them. After providing some historical perspective on health promoters in chapter 1, along with guidance on how to assess health studies, I devote each succeeding chapter to a different area of prevention and a particular type of health seller that is a major force in that area. For example, chapter 2 looks at how the news media, our primary source of information about nutrition, uncritically report industry-funded research and overstate the health benefits of particular foods. Chapter 5 explores how a huge government health campaign, which has been instrumental in shaping our society's agenda on cholesterol, relays oversimplified messages that don't apply equally to everyone. Chapter 8 examines how consumer activists, who have led the way in raising awareness of environmental hazards, cause undue alarm over dangers from chemicals and distort our health priorities.

As you read in these and other chapters about some of the surprising ways we're being spun, note that the methods and motives from each example apply to more than that particular area of health. For instance, the news media regularly rely on industry-backed information for stories regarding not only food but also pharmaceuticals, dietary supplements, and weight loss products.

Also keep in mind that most areas of prevention typically have multiple sellers offering similar advice. I limit my focus in each chapter to one health topic and one type of health promoter in order to illustrate how various players operate to influence us. While each example represents just a slice of reality, I hope that, taken together, these slices give you a comprehensive picture of the health promotion industry—who's part of it, what drives various players, how they present information, and, most important, how you can think more critically about what they tell you.

Though I comment throughout the book on the credibility of specific claims, my real aim is to help you make such determinations for yourself. To that end, each chapter concludes with a list of trustworthy sources of information—science-based, spin-free books, newsletters, and Web sites you can consult to check out specific claims or learn more.

My intention is not to provide an A to Z encyclopedia of prevention and wellness. Plenty of topics that would appear in such a guide, ranging from smoking to vaccinations, are not addressed here. Instead, I have chosen issues that I think best illustrate the workings of the health promotion industry. In discussing them, I've tried to cite the most current science at the time of this writing. But because the field of prevention is constantly evolving, it's possible that by the time you read this, some of what I've written may be superseded by new information.

One more caveat: I've restricted my focus to individual behavior choices—things you can do (or not do) to try to stay healthy. Many public health experts will tell you there's much more to prevention than this. Our environment—and by that I mean not only our air and water but also various social and economic forces—helps determine how healthy we are. Some in public health argue that there's too much emphasis on personal responsibility. Instead, they say, the priority should be to create societal conditions that are more conducive to good health. For example, rather than just urging people to eat better and exercise more, they push to make healthful foods more affordable and communities more exercise-friendly.

By focusing exclusively on individual behavior choices, I don't mean to imply that environmental and social forces don't matter. I'm simply trying to respond to reality. For better or worse, there's a growing push for people to take personal responsibility for their health, a trend fueled by the rise of "consumer-driven" health care and pressures to contain health costs (though not everyone agrees that prevention ultimately saves money). Millions are trying mightily to follow the advice they get from the health promotion industry. My goal is to help us do so more intelligently.

CYNICISM VERSUS SKEPTICISM

None of us wants to be gullible, of course. But as we try to avoid being duped, we also have to be careful not to fall prey to cynicism—the belief that all health promoters are either liars or fools and that we shouldn't listen to any of them. That's not the truth, and it's certainly not the message I want you to take away from this book.

Plenty of health promoters whom I take to task also provide sound information that can potentially benefit your health. That's why you'll see, for example, consumer activists criticized in one chapter but commended in another. It's easy to demonize entire groups—whether drug companies, government agencies, or journalists—and automatically dismiss anything they say. Some who fancy themselves skeptics, including many inhabitants of the blogosphere, have such a mind-set. But they're not really skeptics; they're cynics.

A healthy skeptic carefully and critically evaluates each piece of advice, taking into account not only its source but also the science behind it. Unquestionably, that demands more from us than cynicism does. As Dr. Marcia Angell, a former editor-in-chief of the *New England Journal of Medicine*, has observed: "Cynicism is much easier than skepticism because it requires no distinctions. We needn't distinguish between reliable evidence and unreliable evidence, between big dangers and small ones, between likely effects and unlikely ones, between the reasonable and the bizarre. Yielding to cynicism over skepticism is therefore an easy way out."

Being either gullible or cynical can negatively affect our health. By believing everything—or nothing—we hear, we may fail to take the right steps to stay healthy. There's no question that measures such as exercising, eating a healthful diet, wearing a seat belt, getting vaccinated, not smoking, and not drinking in excess can reduce the risk of illness, injury, and premature death. Indeed, how we live can have a great impact on overall health and longevity. The CDC estimates that more than one-third of all U.S. deaths are attributable to unhealthful behaviors. It's therefore imperative that we, both as individuals and as a society, take prevention seriously and make sure our actions are driven by the best information we can get. Too much is at stake to let ourselves succumb to cynicism or be swayed by spin.

As a health journalist, I'm inundated every day with pitches from all kinds of sellers trying to get their messages across. Some of their ideas are clearly worthwhile; others are downright crazy. The majority fall somewhere in between. Having to sort through this cacophony of claims forces me to draw daily on that lesson I learned long ago from know-it-all Marty: verify before you buy what's being sold. Being a healthy skeptic has not only made me a better journalist, I believe, but also allowed me to make better decisions regarding my own health and given me confidence that I'm on the right track. It's my hope that this book can help do the same for you.

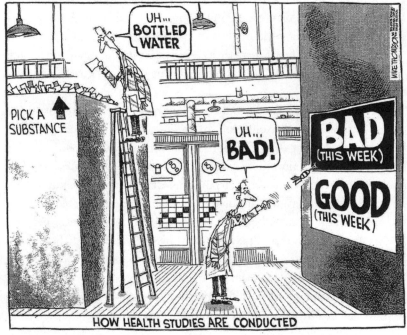

Copley News Service/Mike Thompson

HOW WE KNOW WHAT (WE THINK) WE KNOW

I n the film *The Road to Wellville*, Anthony Hopkins plays Dr. John Harvey Kellogg, the legendary health promoter whose surname is now synonymous with cereal. The doctor, portrayed as a buck-toothed, bowel-obsessed fanatic who pushes daily enemas as the antidote to just about everything, brags (if that's the right word) that "my own stools . . . are gigantic and have no more odor than a hot biscuit."

Adapted from the satiric novel of the same name, the movie shows patients at Dr. Kellogg's Battle Creek Sanitarium engaged in all kinds of bizarre practices, including rhythmic laughing, exercising in diapers, and sitting in electrically charged tubs of water. (In the process, one patient dies of electrocution.) The scenes, fictional but not far from reality, poke fun at Kellogg's silly ideas and the gullibility of so many people, desperately seeking good health, who embraced them.

Though the film's entertainment value is debatable—the movie is filled with bathroom humor and flopped at the box office—its lessons about health promotion are profound. It reminds us of how far we've come in our quest for wellness and, in many ways, how little some things have changed.

One notable difference is the rationale for health recommendations. In previous eras, appeals for healthy living were based on religion, morality, pseudoscience, anecdotal observations, or the personal experiences of health promoters. Today, in contrast, health advice is typically attributed to a seemingly more objective and sophisticated source: modern scientific research.

While not infallible, it can nevertheless be a powerful tool—unavailable to our ancestors—that helps us discern what's true and what's not.

But too often, health promoters misuse, misrepresent, or disregard research altogether, and we unquestioningly accept what we're told, just as Dr. Kellogg's followers did. If you need evidence of this, look no further than the *New York Times* best-seller list. One of the most popular health books in recent memory is *Natural Cures "They" Don't Want You to Know About*, by Kevin Trudeau, a TV infomercial huckster who has been sued by the federal government for making bogus claims and has served prison time for credit card fraud. Though he assures us that "there are more than 900 studies proving the basis [*sic*] premises in this book," his chapter on prevention, titled "How to Never Get Sick Again," includes a smorgasbord of scientifically unsubstantiated directives. Among them: get your colon irrigated; eat bee pollen; sleep on a magnetic mattress pad; don't use deodorant; avoid air conditioning; throw away your microwave oven; stay away from clothes dryers; don't eat for up to a month; and use a machine that "rebalances" your bodily energy.

When we fall for flapdoodle like this, there's little to separate us from those misguided souls in *The Road to Wellville* at whom we laugh. The joke, it seems, is on us. But by gaining some basic knowledge of research and applying a little critical thinking to what we're told, we have the power to keep history from repeating itself.

HEALTH PROMOTION HISTORY HIGHLIGHTS

For some perspective on where we find ourselves today, it's helpful to take a brief look at some health promoters of the past, many of them colorful characters like Kellogg who attracted large followings. As you read through this history of human folly (and occasional wisdom), note the parallels with many modern-day teachings as well as the changes over the centuries in how health promoters have justified their ideas.

ANCIENT WISDOM AND PERSONAL EXPERIENCE

Our journey begins nearly 2,500 years ago with the physician Hippocrates (ca. 460 BC–ca. 377 BC), who recognized and wrote about the influence of diet, exercise, and environmental factors on health. The Greek physician Galen (AD 129–ca. 199), heavily influenced by Hippocrates, formally codified rules for healthful living, which required attention to six "nonnaturals," as they became known: air; motion and rest; sleep and waking; food and drink; excretions; and passions and emotions. In all areas, moderation was key.

These principles continued to hold sway in the mid-sixteenth century, when the Italian nobleman Luigi Cornaro (ca. 1466–1566) wrote a widely circulated series of essays on wellness and longevity, *Discourses on the Sober Life*. The author, who penned the works in his 80s and 90s, tells how he had previously led an indulgent lifestyle that nearly killed him at age 40. In what might be described as a Renaissance version of *Extreme Makeover*, he then adopted a regimen based on the nonnaturals, strictly limiting his consumption of food and wine and avoiding extreme heat and cold, fatigue, and bad air. Adhering to such rules, Cornaro claimed, gave him physical strength, mental clarity, and inner peace as well as immunity to all diseases.

Invoking the "eminent physician" Galen, Cornaro called himself a "living witness" to the truth of the doctor's teachings. He pointed to his own experience as proof that everyone—even those with a "bad constitution"— could avoid illness and infirmity through proper living. He even promised that anyone who followed his example could live to at least 100—a milestone he achieved himself, give or take a few years. (Accounts of his exact age at death vary.)

Similar rationales were prominent in the writings of George Cheyne (1671–1743), an obese Scottish physician who became famous, ironically, for his diet advice. His popular manual *An Essay of Health and Long Life*, first published in 1724 and reprinted in multiple editions and languages, was organized according to Galen's principles, with each chapter corresponding to a different nonnatural. In extolling the virtues of moderation, Cheyne also rooted his advice in the ancient philosophy of Aristotle, who advocated the golden mean, or nothing in excess. "If men would but observe the golden mean in all their passions, appetites, and desires," Cheyne wrote, "they would enjoy a greater measure of health than they do . . . live with less pain, and die with less horror."

Echoing Cornaro, Cheyne cited personal experience as another basis for his recommendations, informing his readers that "I have consulted nothing but my own experience and observation on my own crazy carcass." His carcass tipped the scales at 450 pounds, and Cheyne suffered from repeated bouts of physical and psychological ailments. He recovered (eventually dropping to a svelte 300 pounds) after adopting a relatively spartan diet similar to the one he recommended.

"TRUST ME, I'M A DOCTOR"

But Cheyne also justified his advice in another way: as a physician, he claimed to have an expert understanding of the body's inner workings. Heavily influenced by the natural philosophy of Isaac Newton, Cheyne envisioned the body as a hydraulic machine that could be understood through mathematical calculations. He believed that the machine consisted of pipes, or "canals," through which juices flowed and that keeping the liquids thin and moving was "the great secret of health and long life." Thick and gooey juices supposedly led to disease and death.

Based on these notions, Cheyne offered a contemporary rationale for Galen's ancient rules. For example, he recommended against oily, fatty foods and those with strong odors and tastes because, he reasoned, their particles stuck together more readily and thickened the fluids. Likewise, Cheyne wrote that exercise was essential for keeping the juices flowing. He was especially partial to horseback riding, which he said was capable of "shaking the whole machine, promoting a universal perspiration and secretion of all the fluids." Even though he had no empirical evidence to support his ideas, Cheyne assured readers that his notions had been confirmed through "infinite experiment, and the best natural philosophy."

Medical authority was also the basis for advice in the first U.S. consumer health periodical, which debuted in 1829. Called the *Journal of Health* and edited by "an Association of Physicians" (which actually consisted of just two doctors), the twice-monthly publication focused on "air, food, exercise, the reciprocal action of body and mind, climate and localities, clothing, and the physical education of children." The authors, influenced by the French medical theorist François Broussais, believed that irritation of the stomach— which supposedly could result from overstimulating foods, beverages, emotions, or exertion—lay at the root of virtually all medical conditions. Thus they recommended a plain diet of fruit, vegetables, and breads, along with small amounts of meat. Cleanliness and moderate exercise were in; tobacco and extreme emotions were out.

The *Journal of Health* began during the presidency of Andrew Jackson, an era characterized by rising democratic participation and declining deference to elite authority. That authority included the medical profession, which at the time lacked real cures and instead prescribed ineffective (and sometimes deadly) measures like bloodletting, vomiting, purging, and administering toxic substances such as mercury. Many people, wisely leery of such treatments, were turning instead to alternatives, including botanical healing, homeopathy, and self-care. The journal's editors, trying to stem this tide, denounced such practices and stressed the essential role of the trained physician—whom they called the "only competent judge" of disease. Apparently, this was a message the public didn't want to hear: four years after its launch, the *Journal of Health* went out of business.

GOD'S LAWS

About the same time, Sylvester Graham (1794–1851), most often remembered as the grandfather of the Graham cracker, was rising to prominence. A Presbyterian minister and gifted orator who began his career giving anti-alcohol lectures, he soon broadened his focus to health habits. Unlike the editors of the *Journal of Health*, Graham was not part of the medical establishment and made no attempt to defend it. In fact, he was disdainful of doctors, declaring that "all medicine, as such, is itself an evil."

While others before him had invoked God's laws as a source of their ideas, Graham went further, turning health promotion into a moral crusade. He taught that by living temperate lives according to God's laws of health—rules that just so happened to coincide with God's moral laws—human beings could achieve physical perfection, create heaven on earth, and hasten the Second Coming of Christ. It was a "morally binding duty," Graham's disciples believed, to study and obey the laws "which God has established for the perpetuation of [humankind's] existence."

Under Graham's principles of disease prevention, which he called "the Science of Human Life," just about everything considered immoral was now deemed unhealthful—and that included sex. Warning that sexual excess caused debilitation, he advised healthy married couples to limit their sexual activity to once a month. Sex outside marriage was even more injurious, he reasoned, because it was more exciting. Worst of all was masturbation because it involved the imagination and therefore inflamed the brain, leading to insanity.

Graham claimed that exercise could keep sexual urges in check, as could a nonstimulating diet, which he recommended for everyone. Meat was forbidden, as were mustard, pepper, soups, cream, butter, pastries, tea, and coffee. Graham had special contempt for store-bought white bread, as he believed that stripping bran from flour rendered bread overly stimulating. Instead, he extolled the health virtues of old-fashioned, homemade bread baked with whole-grain flour—what became known as "Graham flour." (Ironically, leading brands of Graham crackers are today manufactured with the type of refined flour Graham abhorred.)

Graham stopped lecturing in 1839, but his cause continued under the leadership of Dr. William Alcott (1798–1859), a prolific author of advice manuals for both adults and young people. Alcott's message generally mirrored that of Graham, though he went even further in portraying himself as a "medical missionary" who was spreading God's gospel of health. For example, defending the idea that people should restrict themselves to monthly sex, he acknowledged that the stricture was unpopular and seemed "rigid." But, he asked rhetorically, "Am I at fault, in announcing it? I certainly *did* not *make* the law. At most, I am but its interpreter." He was, like Moses, simply revealing God's laws.

At the same time, Alcott tried to debunk the popular notion that sickness and death were God's will. "It is much easier, or at least much lazier," he wrote, "to refer all our ills and complaints, as well as their unfavorable terminations, to God or Satan . . . than to consider [ourselves] as the probable cause." This idea of human control over health—that it was possible, indeed obligatory, for human beings to achieve perfect health—was central to Graham's ideology. It grew out of a larger American phenomenon of the early nineteenth century, the Second Great Awakening, a revivalist movement that challenged the Calvinist concept of helpless human beings whose destiny was entirely up to God. Instead, evangelists preached, people had the power and the duty to eliminate the evils they faced—including disease—and thereby achieve salvation.

GOD SPEAKS

Another product of the Second Great Awakening was the Seventh-Day Adventists, a religious group that focused on preparing for Christ's Second Coming. Its leader, Ellen White (1827–1915), stressed the importance of following God's laws of health, teaching that violating them was akin to breaking the Ten Commandments. But unlike Graham and Alcott, who had become aware of such laws through books, intuition, or observation, White announced that she had been enlightened directly by the Lord.

In a series of "visions"—trancelike experiences in which she claimed to see angels, Jesus, and Satan—White supposedly learned that tobacco, tea, coffee, meat, butter, eggs, cheese, rich foods, and uncleanliness, among other things, were harmful. In her writings and lectures, she often gave physiological explanations for the rules God had revealed to her. For example, she wrote that meat was hazardous because it transmitted disease and stirred up animal passions.

Though White insisted her views had come from God and were "independent of books or of the opinion of others," her pronouncements bore a striking resemblance to those of Graham, Alcott, and other like-minded health promoters. She appeared to borrow especially heavily from a physician and preacher named Larkin Coles, the author of a popular health advice manual, *Philosophy of Health*. An analysis of White's writings by historian Ronald Numbers reveals how she frequently lifted passages almost verbatim from Coles's work without attribution.

White was also influenced by James Jackson, who ran a health facility in Dansville, New York, known as Our Home on the Hillside. There, Jackson combined Graham's health regimen with hydropathy, an unorthodox healing method using water as a cure-all. After visiting Our Home, White had a vision that Adventists should establish their own health institution. In 1866, the Western Health Reform Institute (later renamed the Battle Creek Sanitarium) opened its doors in Battle Creek, Michigan.

SELECTIVE SCIENCE

A decade later, White tapped then 24-year-old Dr. John Harvey Kellogg (1852–1943) to head the institute. He would remain there for 67 years and would become, in the words of medical historian James Whorton, "the most formidable reformer of American living habits of the twentieth century." During the doctor's long career, medicine would experience remarkable progress, becoming a true science. Unlike White, who had no use for orthodox medicine, Kellogg embraced it, even boasting that he was years ahead of other doctors in incorporating the latest ideas and practices. But in reality, he did so selectively, adopting only those theories that he could apply—or twist—to lend credence to his preconceived notions.

Kellogg, the son of a devout Adventist, was first drawn to those notions as a teenager. As an apprentice typesetter for White's husband, James, who ran the Adventists' publications division, Kellogg worked on a series of health advice pamphlets that included writings by Ellen White, Sylvester Graham, and others. Intrigued at what he read, he delved further into the works of Graham in his spare time and became a vegetarian.

Sent to medical school by the Whites, he found that many of the ideas he'd been exposed to under their tutelage were considered nonsense by mainstream doctors. Still, Kellogg clung tenaciously to those beliefs, forming bonds with professors whose ideas were compatible with his own.

It was a pattern that continued throughout his entire career: Kellogg looked to modern medical science to validate the dogma passed down to him from White and Graham. To lend his old ideas an air of scientific legitimacy, he gave them a new name, "biologic living." And he latched on to any scientific theory that might somehow support his cause. For example, he readily adopted the germ theory as it was just starting to gain acceptance and used it to further his arguments against eating meat. In one "experiment," he "proved" that beefsteak contained more harmful germs than barnyard manure.

Likewise, Kellogg championed the theory of a Russian zoologist who argued that bacteria from decaying protein in the colon entered the bloodstream and "poisoned" the body. Kellogg attributed this phenomenon, known as autointoxication, to eating meat and claimed that it caused a wide range of conditions, including skin problems, depression, and liver damage. The solution consisted of a high-fiber, vegetable diet, combined with colon irrigation to promote multiple daily bowel movements.

In his writings, Kellogg often cited the opinions of other physicians to bolster his ideas, including his draconian views on sex. For example, his sex and marriage manual quoted several "eminent" and "learned" medical authorities to make the case that too much marital sex could be harmful, leading to everything from sore throats to consumption. But his harshest denunciations were aimed at masturbation, which he called "the most dangerous of all sexual abuses." As evidence, Kellogg cited the "testimony of eminent authors," one of whom opined that "neither the plague, nor war, nor small-pox, nor similar diseases, have produced results so disastrous to humanity as the pernicious habit."

To head off this horror, Kellogg invoked yet another so-called expert, Dr. O.W. Archibald, superintendent of the Iowa Asylum for Feeble-Minded Children, who recommended sewing the foreskin shut over the penis in order to make an erection impossible. Another suggested remedy, which Kellogg described as "almost always successful in small boys," was performing a circumcision—without anesthesia. For female offenders, he recommended applying acid to the clitoris, which he found to be "an excellent means of allaying . . . abnormal excitement." Apparently with a straight face, Kellogg denounced other (presumably less severe) anti-masturbation measures as scientifically unsound, warning readers to beware of "pretentious quacks" who offered them.

Bolstering Kellogg's claims to being on the cutting edge of science were his numerous inventions, which included everything from surgical instruments to meat substitutes. But his most famous creation was ready-to-eat, flaked cereal, which he developed with his brother Will. (Eventually, Will formed his own cereal business, which became the Kellogg Company that exists today.)

Through the force of his personality and his penchant for self-promotion, Dr. Kellogg managed to gain enormous fame and respect as a medical authority, despite his selective use of science. During his long career, he wrote nearly 50 books, edited a magazine called *Good Health*, and gave thousands of lectures across the country to both professional and lay audiences. Over the years, his Battle Creek Sanitarium (or the "San," as it was known) attracted the rich and famous, including Henry Ford, Thomas Edison, and Amelia Earhart, among its more than 300,000 guests.

A name surely familiar to visitors at the San after the turn of the century was Horace Fletcher (1849–1919), known as "the Great Masticator." A friend of Kellogg's, Fletcher championed the notion that the secret to health was chewing food until it liquefied. Declaring that Fletcher "had done more to help suffering humanity than any other man of the present generation," Kellogg was so taken with Fletcher's ideas that he wrote a "Chewing Song" for his patients and coined the term "Fletcherize," meaning to chew thoroughly.

A successful businessman and former athlete, Fletcher found himself tired, sick, and obese at age 40. After adopting his chewing regimen, he dropped more than 50 pounds within four months and lost 7 inches off his waist. His ailments and fatigue vanished. To spread the word about his remarkable success, he wrote, lectured, gave press interviews, and offered public demonstrations of his vigor, which included backward flips off a diving board, lifting a man on his shoulders, and cycling 190 miles.

Fletcher used his considerable wealth not only to market his health secret but also to buy credibility from the medical establishment. To scientifically test his theory, he funded "studies" at Yale on his own physical fitness. In one, the investigator concluded that the 54-year-old Fletcher had performed "with greater ease and with fewer noticeable bad results than any man of his age and condition I have ever worked with."

Fletcher's explanation was that his interminable chewing prevented solid, decaying wastes from accumulating in his digestive tract and poisoning his body. But for the Yale nutrition expert overseeing the studies, the issue wasn't Fletcher's chewing but the fact that his subject had (unwittingly) reduced his protein intake. Further studies, some funded by Fletcher, would eventually lead experts to lower their protein recommendations. In such a way, Fletcher had a lasting impact on science. But the practice of Fletcherizing, despite the popularity and buzz generated by its inventor, died when he did.

ALTERNATIVE "SCIENCE"

Unlike Kellogg and Fletcher, the popular bodybuilding enthusiast Bernarr Macfadden (1868–1955) didn't look to the medical establishment for validation. Instead, he vociferously attacked it, calling it "the science of guessing" that belonged "to the ignorance of the distant past." Believing that germs didn't pose a threat to healthy people—he privately called Louis Pasteur, the father of the germ theory, "that French quack"—Macfadden strongly opposed vaccines as well as the use of medications and surgery. He accused doctors, especially leaders of the American Medical Association, of being liars and phonies who cared most about their own financial interests.

Macfadden's alternative to medicine was his self-invented science, which he called physcultopathy. Citing his own experiences and those of others to support his theories, he argued that all diseases stemmed from impurity in the blood and that they could be prevented or cured through proper living. That meant a regimen similar to Kellogg's and Graham's, except that Macfadden was not a vegetarian, and he put special emphasis on regular fasting as a way to eliminate poisons from the body.

The Macfadden wellness regimen was also novel in its emphasis on fitness and strength over everything else—something reflected in the title of Macfadden's highly popular magazine, *Physical Culture*, and in its motto: "Weakness is a crime; don't be a criminal." Beautiful bodies (often displayed scantily clad or nude) were a sign of not only perfect health, he argued, but also strong character. Having changed his birth name of Bernard McFadden to one he thought sounded more powerful, he relentlessly promoted his own perfectly sculpted physique and vitality as firsthand evidence for his theories.

An outlandish and irrepressible showman, Macfadden was a master marketer of his cause. Like other health promoters of his era, he wrote prolifically to promote his ideas, authoring or editing almost 150 books and pamphlets, including a multivolume *Encyclopedia of Physical Culture*. He was also a frequent contributor to *Physical Culture* magazine, just one of many publications he owned.

FROM BELIEFS TO EVIDENCE

J. I. Rodale (1898–1971), an accountant turned farmer, publisher, and health promoter, considered Macfadden his hero. Like Macfadden, Rodale had his own set of idiosyncratic health beliefs, many of which had little or no solid science behind them. And he too pushed his ideas through the books and magazines he published. But unlike Macfadden, Rodale created a publishing empire that outlived him, and his company eventually came to offer advice based on more than just its founder's opinions.

An early advocate of organic farming, Rodale believed that chemical fertilizers and pesticides were harmful to both the environment and human health. Going further, he opposed synthetic chemicals of all kinds and warned about health hazards from food additives, plastic utensils, aluminum cookware, and fluoridated water, among other things. He gave his enthusiastic blessing to "natural" food supplements, for which he often made wildly exaggerated claims: sunflower seeds preserved eyesight; bone meal could prevent both asthma and cavities; magnesium was a "miracle mineral"; and hawthorn berries and vitamin E were "an unbeatable combination to combat heart disease." Rodale himself swallowed as many as a hundred supplements a day, including everything from desiccated liver to dolomite.

Like health promoters before him, Rodale had a fairly lengthy list of forbidden foods. At the top was sugar, which he believed caused antisocial behavior. Milk made people too tall, he believed, and white bread led to colds. He was no fonder of wheat, whether in bread or cereal. Negative emotions were also off-limits, an old principle that Rodale took to new extremes in an article, and later a book, titled "Happy People Rarely Get Cancer."

To reach such conclusions, Rodale frequently cited testimonials from readers and results from so-called experiments he conducted by monitoring himself. But he also read medical journals and cited mainstream research whenever he could to help make his case. Over time, *Prevention* magazine—the highly popular health publication he founded in 1950—would increasingly use this standard as the basis for its advice, moving away from simply promoting the personal beliefs of the company's founder and toward providing more objective and seemingly evidence-based information.

"RESEARCH PROVES ..."

Indeed, most major health promoters today, whether mainstream or not, at least profess to base their recommendations on scientific research. In persuading us to follow particular advice, they typically use phrases like "studies show" or "research proves"—modern-day versions of their predecessors' exhortations "God wants you to do this" or "it worked for me" or simply "trust me." In principle at least, this shift to a more neutral, objective standard is a positive development, taking us out of the realm of faith and belief into that of facts and knowledge.

But if you dig beneath the surface a bit, you'll find that the evidence cited by health promoters doesn't always support their claims. Overstating the strength, certainty, and scope of the science, they may play up studies that are highly preliminary, poorly conducted, or irrelevant, while conveniently ignoring those that contradict their case.

Consider, for example, the popular health promoter Dr. Nicholas Perricone. Through his television appearances and best-selling books (which include *The Perricone Prescription* and *The Perricone Promise*), this celebrity dermatologist peddles the half-baked idea that inflammation is the root of all health evils. The regimen he pushes, which is supposed to make you look younger and live longer, bans a long list of foods, including bananas, grapes, coffee, carrots, peas, popcorn, oranges, raisins, pasta, pickles, and hard cheese. Instead, we're told to eat wild Alaskan salmon—as often as several times a day—and down eight to ten glasses of water (not just any water, but *spring* water) daily. In addition, Perricone recommends taking more than twenty-five supplements, many with tongue-twister names, such as benfotiamine and chromium polynicotinate.

Sound familiar? Elements of Perricone's regimen bear a striking resemblance to the spoutings of Sylvester Graham (good and evil foods), John Harvey Kellogg (a one-size-fits-all theory of disease), and J. I. Rodale (lifesaving supplements). The difference is that Perricone's books are filled with references to research studies, giving his ideas the veneer of scientific legitimacy. But Drs. Harriet Hall and Stephen Barrett of Quackwatch, an organization that exposes health fraud, aren't fooled. Calling Perricone's recommendations a "fanciful interpretation of selected medical literature," they point out that he "cherry picks possibly supportive studies from the literature and ignores contradictory studies. He cites lots of lab studies . . . but few that demonstrate any clinical effects in humans." In short, they write, Perricone "has mixed a pinch of science with a gallon of imagination."

ASSESSING THE SCIENCE

To assess the legitimacy of claims by Perricone and other health promoters, it's important to have at least a basic understanding of how research is conducted and how to interpret findings. When you hear that "studies prove" something to be true, consider the following eight key questions before drawing any conclusions. This assessment may require some digging, and the answers won't always be available, but the extra effort will pay off by empowering you to make smarter decisions about your health.

1. WHAT KIND OF STUDY IS IT?

Much of the research cited by health promoters comes from the field of epidemiology, the study of disease patterns and their contributors in populations. Typically, epidemiological studies are observational, meaning that scientists measure something but don't intervene. While such research can identify probable health risks and benefits, it can't definitively prove cause and effect. Types of observational studies include the following:

> *Population studies.* These usually compare groups in different geographic areas, looking for differences both in disease rates and in some factor or factors (known as exposures) that might be responsible. An example is the so-called Seven Countries Study, which found that nations like Finland, where heart disease rates were relatively high, had higher-fat diets than places like Japan, where heart disease was less common. The research appeared to support the idea that dietary fat caused heart disease. The problem with such studies is that the apparent suspect—in this case, fat—may not be the real culprit. For example, populations who consume less fat might also get more physical activity, eat more fish, or have other related characteristics that may actually account for the lower rates of disease. These extraneous factors, known as confounders, can make population studies—as well as other observational studies—tricky to interpret.

> *Case-control studies.* Researchers select two groups that are similar in all ways except that the members of one (the cases) have the disease in question and the members of the other (the controls) do not. Information is then gathered about the subjects' past habits to find differences

that may explain the occurrence of disease. For example, case-control studies have found that women with bladder cancer are more likely to have used permanent hair dye than those without the disease. While this suggests a possible connection, it is not proof. When asked to recall their habits from years or decades ago, people often have fuzzy memories. Those with the disease who are searching for a cause may remember (or think they remember) things that controls don't. It's also possible that the two groups aren't as similar as the researchers believe. Perhaps the cases are different from the controls in some way, aside from the exposure, that affects their risk of illness.

Cohort studies. These studies, in contrast, are typically forward looking. Healthy people are evaluated for various exposures and then followed for years or decades to see who gets the disease(s) in question and who doesn't. A classic example is the ongoing Framingham Heart Study, begun in 1948. At the start of the study, 5,000 residents of Framingham, Massachusetts, who were free of heart disease were questioned extensively about their lifestyle habits and given tests measuring blood pressure, cholesterol, and other characteristics. Periodically over the following years, information has been updated and tests have been repeated. The study has found, for example, that residents who smoke or have high blood pressure or high cholesterol are more likely to develop heart disease than nonsmokers or those who have normal blood pressure and cholesterol. Though cohort studies are considered more definitive than case-control studies, they too have potential drawbacks. Among other things, keeping track of thousands or tens of thousands of people for many years is a huge challenge, and if enough subjects fall off the radar, it can skew the results.

In contrast to observational investigations, other types of studies involve an intervention by the researcher:

Randomized clinical trials. In these studies, individuals are randomly assigned to receive either the factor being tested (the experimental group) or a fake look-alike called a placebo (the control group). Typically, neither subjects nor researchers know who has been assigned to which group—a practice known as double-blinding. The two groups are then followed for a period of time (sometimes many years) to determine whether they fare differently. Randomized clinical trials can confirm or refute associations revealed by observational studies and provide proof of a cause-and-effect relationship. But even randomized trials aren't foolproof; a flawed study design can produce flawed results. What's more, clinical trials generally are not appropriate for confirming suspected risks, as intentionally exposing people to potential harm would be unethical.

Short-term human studies. Like large clinical trials, these studies may have randomly assigned placebo and control groups. They typically include relatively small numbers of subjects who are exposed to the factor in question. After hours, days, or months, researchers measure some marker, such as the level of a particular substance in the blood, to determine the factor's physiological effects. Many foods and dietary supplements believed to confer health benefits are tested this way. While such research can be valuable by providing hints of an effect on disease, the evidence is generally considered preliminary. That's because demonstrating a short-term change in blood chemistry, for example, is a far cry from showing a change in subjects' rates of disease.

Laboratory research. Studies conducted on animals or on human cells and tissues (so-called test-tube research) can help establish hypotheses about possible risks or benefits that require further investigation in human trials. They can also help corroborate epidemiological findings by providing a biological explanation. What's more, lab research can come in handy when human studies aren't possible or ethical. Its main advantage is that researchers can control exactly what happens, eliminating the impact of extraneous factors that so often plague human experiments. Its disadvantage is that such research may have limited relevance to human beings in the real world. A laboratory rat is not a person, after all, and what causes disease in one may not do so in the other.

In general, here's how the different types of studies rank in terms of the credibility of evidence they produce:

Test-tube research   Least credible
Animal studies
Population studies
Short-term human experiments
Case-control studies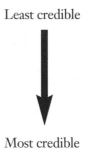
Cohort studies
Randomized clinical trials   Most credible

2. HOW BIG IS THE EFFECT?

Generally, the larger the effect, the more believable it is. In observational studies, an association (typically expressed as a "relative risk") that's strong is less likely than a weak one to be influenced by confounding factors. For example, male smokers are 23 times more likely than male nonsmokers to die from lung cancer. This relative risk of 23 is so large that no extraneous factor can probably account for it. But the same can't be said for the association between breast cancer and alcohol consumption among women. According to one study, the relative risk of breast cancer among post-menopausal women who drink is 1.3—that is, they have a 30 percent greater risk than nondrinkers. (A relative risk of 1.0 means no increase in risk, a relative risk of 2.0 equals a 100 percent greater risk, a relative risk of 3.0 translates into a 200 percent greater risk, and so forth.) That relative risk of 1.3 is so small that it could be partly or completely due to confounders. Broadly speaking, many epidemiologists consider any increase in relative risk under 3 to be relatively small and worthy of extra skepticism, especially if the finding has not been corroborated by other studies.

In addition to knowing the relative increase (or decrease), it's crucial to find out the absolute difference in risk. For example, let's assume that people exposed to substance X have triple the risk of contracting disease Y. At first glance, this may seem scary. But if you also learn that the prevalence of this particular disease is one in a million among unexposed people and three in a million among those who were exposed, there's less reason for concern: the absolute increase in risk is just two cases per million, or .0002 percent. It's an illustration of how the relative risk, viewed in isolation without the absolute numbers, can be highly misleading.

3. COULD THE FINDINGS BE A FLUKE?

Researchers try to determine the validity of their findings through measures of statistical significance—an often-misunderstood concept. In research, the term "significance" doesn't denote importance or size, as it does in everyday use; instead, it refers to the role of chance. When results are statistically significant, there's only a very small probability—typically less than 5 percent—that the findings are a fluke. While this provides some assurance that the outcome was not due to chance, it doesn't rule out the possibility completely, nor does it address whether confounders or other problems may have skewed the results.

4. WHO WAS STUDIED?

To figure out whether findings might apply to you, it's important to consider who was studied. Researchers often study homogeneous populations in order to minimize the possible role of confounding factors. But what's true for healthy college students or middle-aged white men or postmenopausal women may not be so for others. It's therefore important to be careful in extrapolating findings from one group to another.

5. IS THERE A GOOD EXPLANATION?

Findings from observational studies are more credible if there's a known (or at least plausible) biological explanation for them. When studies yield findings that don't make sense biologically, they should be interpreted with great caution, especially when the association is weak and therefore possibly the result of confounding factors.

6. WHO PAID FOR THE RESEARCH?

Many studies are funded by organizations with a vested interest in the outcome, such as drug companies, food producers, dietary supplement manufacturers, or consumer activists. Such sponsorship doesn't necessarily render the findings invalid, but it does raise the possibility that the study's methods or conclusions were either directly or indirectly influenced by the funder's agenda. Research supported by more neutral entities such as the Centers for Disease Control and Prevention or the National Institutes of Health is therefore sometimes considered more credible.

7. WAS IT PEER REVIEWED?

To determine whether a research paper is worthy of publication, most journals—though not all—subject it to the scrutiny of outside experts, who dissect the methodology and the author's interpretations. Although this process by no means guarantees that a study is flawless (plenty of questionable ones make it through peer review), it does add an extra layer of credibility. Studies are sometimes presented at scientific conferences—and cited by media reports and health promoters—before full peer review and publication. Because many such studies end up never making the cut and getting published, they deserve to be taken less seriously than thoroughly peer-reviewed research. The same goes for industry-conducted research that's shielded from outside evaluation.

8. HOW DOES IT SQUARE WITH OTHER STUDIES?

This is perhaps the most crucial question. Rarely is any study, by itself, definitive. Instead, each is a piece of a puzzle. Only when a sufficient number of pieces have been assembled does a clear picture emerge. That's why interpreting a study requires knowing how it fits with others that came before it. How does it add to what's already known? Is it consistent with previous findings? If it conflicts, why? To get to the truth, it's necessary to examine the research as a whole—what scientists call the totality of the evidence. Viewing a study in isolation, like seeing just one piece of a puzzle, can give an erroneous impression.

SHADES OF GRAY

Getting answers to these eight questions can go a long way toward helping you determine the credibility and relevance of a health claim. But it's not as simple as plugging your responses into a formula and calculating the final answer. Figuring out what to make of a study—or a series of studies—and how to respond is still a judgment call. For most issues, we don't have large, randomized clinical trials that provide incontrovertible evidence, so we have to make decisions based on something less. Part of being a healthy skeptic is understanding that studies, when honestly interpreted, don't always produce the definitive "yes or no" answers we'd like.

This can certainly be frustrating. Throughout this book, you'll repeatedly encounter less than conclusive statements such as "studies suggest" this or "there's little evidence" of that. You'll also see references to areas of research in which some studies show one thing, while others show the opposite—the classic "coffee is bad for you . . . wait, it's good . . . no, it's bad" flip-flops we so often encounter. If you're tempted to respond by throwing up your hands and saying, "I give up," remember that changing how you think about health information, which is necessary to becoming a healthy skeptic, takes time and patience. Rather than demanding black and white answers, we have to learn to live with, and distinguish among, various shades of gray.

How much gray is acceptable can differ depending on the issue and the individual. For example, to justify taking preventive medication such as hormone replacement therapy, a healthy woman might rightly look for ironclad evidence of considerable benefits that greatly outweigh any risks. But when faced with a potential hazard, she may have a somewhat lower burden of proof, opting to act before there's an absolutely airtight case. After all, no one wants to repeat the mistake of those (including some doctors) who for years refused to accept that smoking caused cancer because it hadn't been definitively proven. Whatever the circumstance, however, a healthy skeptic doesn't jump to premature conclusions based on evidence that's preliminary, weak, or nonexistent.

Recognizing that most people don't like ambiguity, health promoters sometimes give us simplistic pronouncements—"blueberries fight cancer," "high cholesterol is a killer," "this test will save your life"—that don't convey the full truth. Instead of balanced assessments of science, which is what we need to make informed decisions, we get dogmatic decrees.

When we unquestioningly accept such advice, we're hardly more enlightened (despite our illusions to the contrary) than previous generations who didn't have the benefit of research. If we're told that walnuts will ward off illness, and we believe it without really understanding the evidence, are we any more savvy than the followers of Sylvester Graham who put their faith in whole flour simply because he (or God) told them to? If we believe that cosmetics will give us cancer without scrutinizing the scientific basis for such a claim, are we much different from the disciples of John Harvey Kellogg who believed, based on his assurances, that sex would do them in?

By giving us the unprecedented ability to separate beliefs from facts, scientific research represents the best hope we have—and have ever had—for determining what really helps and harms our health. It can make us smarter than our ancestors, but only if we, as healthy skeptics, put it to proper use.

TRUSTWORTHY SOURCES OF INFORMATION

PubMed (www.pubmed.gov), a service of the U.S National Library of Medicine. PubMed allows you to search for just about any published health or medical article according to topic, author, or journal. You can get abstracts, and in some cases entire articles, free of charge.

The Cochrane Collaboration (www.cochrane.org). A highly respected organization that reviews and summarizes evidence on a variety of health issues.

Health News Review (www.healthnewsreview.org). This award-winning Web site evaluates the accuracy, balance, and completeness of news reports about research findings.

Know Your Chances: Understanding Health Statistics, by Steven Woloshin, Lisa Schwartz, and H. Gilbert Welch (Berkeley: University of California Press, 2008). This is an informative, easy-to-understand guide on interpreting information about health risks and benefits.

Quackwatch (www.quackwatch.org), a group whose mission is to "combat health-related frauds, myths, fads, fallacies, and misconduct." Its Web site includes detailed analyses of numerous questionable claims.

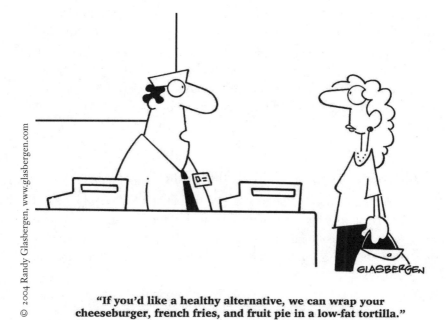

© 2004 Randy Glasbergen, www.glasbergen.com

"If you'd like a healthy alternative, we can wrap your
cheeseburger, french fries, and fruit pie in a low-fat tortilla."

CHAPTER TWO: THE NEWS MEDIA
EAT THIS!

O f all the reasons I decided to become a health journalist, being popular at parties was not among them. It never dawned on me that immersing myself in topics such as the latest remedies for hemorrhoids or the chief causes of foot fungus would endear me to strangers. Yet I've found, much to my surprise, that it often does. As soon as people learn what I do for a living, they frequently corner me and start firing away with questions about some health-related issue. And by far the most common issue is nutrition.

Whether the questioners are strangers, friends, relatives, or readers, they usually want to know which foods are bad for them, which are good, and which they should be eating more regularly. One friend went so far as to ask me via e-mail to list the ten most healthful foods so he could stock up on them. When I replied that instead of fixating on particular foods, he would be better off focusing on his overall diet and exercising, he wasn't satisfied. "Why not try to create a personal diet that includes foods that studies show best promote health?" he replied. "Every little bit helps."

This friend is no fool; he's one of the smartest people I know. Yet, like many others, he's fallen for what I call the superfood fallacy: the unproven notion that specific foods, in isolation, have the power to head off heart disease, cancer, and other conditions. While the appeal of this idea is evident—who can resist the allure of a life-prolonging bowl of berries, after all?—the way it's being peddled isn't always so obvious. The food industry, using science and the news media in sophisticated behind-the-scenes marketing efforts, is successfully spinning us, and in many cases we don't even realize it. The U.S. Food and Drug Administration (FDA), which regulates food claims on labels, is of only limited help in keeping companies honest. It's no surprise, then, that even the most astute among us can be sold on the power of superfoods.

SCIENCE MEETS MARKETING

The relationship between food and health is notoriously complex and difficult to study. Yet multiple studies over several decades have produced fairly solid evidence that certain broad categories of foods, including fruits, vegetables, whole grains, fish, and legumes, may be beneficial.

In recent years, there's been an explosion of research on particular substances in these and other foods—everything from alpha-linolenic acid to zeaxanthin—that might account for the foods' healthfulness. Though this line of inquiry is interesting scientifically, it's still by and large in its infancy. Because foods contain multiple nutrients, which may interact with one another and with other foods to affect our bodies in myriad ways, teasing out the precise effects of a single constituent in one food is tricky business, to say the least. Consequently, the research is not easily translated (at least responsibly so) into specific dietary recommendations. But that hasn't stopped the food industry from using it to promote the idea that so-called superfoods contain magical ingredients capable of warding off illness.

Take, for example, tomatoes. They and their derivatives, such as tomato juice, spaghetti sauce, and ketchup, have been touted by industry as disease fighters because they contain lycopene, an antioxidant that some research has linked to lower rates of prostate and other cancers. (Antioxidants are substances thought to fight free radicals, which can damage cells and thereby cause disease.) Not to be outdone, watermelon growers have promoted their fruit as the "lycopene leader," pointing out that watermelon contains more lycopene than tomatoes. Never mind that the evidence on lycopene and cancer is far from conclusive—not all studies have found a link—and no one knows for certain how much lycopene, if any, is beneficial.

Yet the implicit message is that by eating an extra slice of pizza or watermelon here and there, we'll help protect ourselves against disease. Indeed, the H. J. Heinz Company, which dubs itself "the industry leader in lycopene education and information," comes pretty close to saying this explicitly. Under the slogan "Small Changes, Big Benefits," the company pushes the idea—the one expressed by my friend in his e-mail—that every little bit helps our health. Putting this principle into practice, it provides a recipe using Heinz ketchup as an ingredient in, of all things, cookies. These particular cookies, we're told, are "an easy and tasty way to incorporate more lycopene into the diet." (The amount of lycopene is a minuscule 0.6 mg per cookie.)

It would be nice if adding a little ketchup to our cookies protected us from cancer. Unfortunately, though, it's unproven that tinkering with our diets like this really reduces our susceptibility to disease or premature death. Tossing some blueberries into a cup of ice cream may make us feel more virtuous, and throwing a tomato onto a burger may lessen our guilt over eating those fries that came with it. But in the long run, what matters, according to research, is our overall diet—not whether we include one specific food or another.

SUPERFOOD NEWS

The concept of superfoods is often promoted through consumer health books, whose over-the-top titles tout "miracle foods," "vitality foods," or "miracle superfoods." Though their lists of foods may differ, the books tend to make similarly overblown promises—to "heal the body and mind," "turn back the clock," or "change your life," for example. Not that there's anything wrong with most of these recommended foods; they tend to represent various categories (such as fruits, vegetables, lean meats, nuts, fish) that solid research has shown to be components of a healthful diet. The problem is that the authors, some of whom have advanced degrees in medicine or nutrition, overstate the evidence, drawing definitive conclusions—blueberries prevent Alzheimer's disease; pumpkin protects against cancer; tea guards against hip fractures—from preliminary research, much of it conducted only in test tubes or on animals. In many cases, these books do offer sound advice about eating a healthful diet overall, but you have to wade through lots of scientifically shaky superfood superlatives to get it.

By far the biggest purveyors of the superfood fallacy are the news media, which frequently report on new research suggesting that a particular food may prevent or treat illness. The headlines are attention-grabbing:

"Beans and Soy May Help Prevent Lung Cancer"
"Onions Could Be Good for the Bones"
"Raisins May Help Fight Cavities"
"Sauerkraut Packed with Cancer-Fighting Compounds"
"Alfalfa Could Fight Vision Loss"

And the main message of these stories is irresistible: that simply adding a bit of this or that to our diet can preserve our health and even save our lives. Since we get most of our nutrition-related information from the news media, such coverage unquestionably shapes how we think about food and health.

We have little reason to doubt such reports. After all, they typically involve research conducted by independent scientists, sometimes at well-known universities, and are relayed by journalists at mainstream news organizations, which, we assume, have no financial incentive to hawk particular foods. Reporters are simply passing along the latest scientific findings, it seems.

If only it were that simple. The truth is that stories like these are often the result of back-door marketing campaigns funded by industry and orchestrated by public relations professionals. These sophisticated spin efforts skillfully use science to lend credibility to industry's messages and use journalists to serve as the messengers. Simply put, here's how the process often works:

Step 1: A food manufacturer or trade group funds research conducted by a university scientist.

Step 2: The researcher discovers that a food appears to confer health benefits and presents the findings at a scientific conference or publishes them in a journal.

Step 3: Public relations spinmeisters, hired by industry, issue a press release or other report to the media that trumpets the findings and exaggerates their importance.

Step 4: Adopting the tone or even the exact wording of the industry's public relations materials, journalists craft stories that portray the food as a magic bullet and the findings as conclusive.

Step 5: We buy and eat more of the particular food.

Corporate funding of nutrition research, which is increasingly common, enables scientists to conduct studies that might not otherwise be possible. Most researchers who accept such money will tell you it has no influence over their work. As one scientist put it, "You'd have to be a fool—and a career-ending fool—to let your funding source dictate your results." That may be true, but some evidence suggests that there's at least a correlation between corporate sponsorship and research outcomes. In one study, researchers whose findings or opinions reflected favorably on the fat substitute olestra were far more likely to have financial ties to olestra's manufacturer than scientists whose findings were neutral or unfavorable. Likewise, an analysis of studies on soft drinks, juices, and milk found that those funded by industry were more likely to report positive results for the sponsor than those without industry funding. To most of us, none of this is too surprising because, in the words of nutrition researcher and author Marion Nestle, "it seems counter-intuitive to think that companies would sponsor studies likely to produce unfavorable results."

Scientists are often under enormous pressure to bring in research money, which they need to survive professionally. Consequently, there's a natural tendency to want to keep funders happy, which can manifest itself in subtle ways. For example, researchers may formulate a hypothesis or design an experiment in a manner that's most likely to show benefits for a food. They may frame the data to make those benefits appear as large as possible. Or they may selectively publish data that reflect most favorably on the food and keep quiet about findings that don't. Though universities typically have policies to prevent conflicts of interest with industry, one nutrition professor notes that "when the negotiations come down to the wire, and money and jobs are at stake, then a code of conduct may not be enough to keep a researcher on the straight and narrow."

The link between funding and findings may also be explained by corporate funders' tendency to gravitate toward scientists who seem likely, based on their previous research and opinions, to reach conclusions consistent with the funders' aims. For example, a researcher who has repeatedly deemed a particular food or ingredient to be beneficial is likely to keep doing so— especially if it has helped build his or her professional reputation. Such a pattern may lead to research funding from the food's manufacturer, which begets further favorable findings for the industry, which begets more research dollars for the scientist. The cycle continues, with the industry able to point to a "body of evidence" (even though it's mainly from one scientist) supporting its agenda. The scientist enjoys a steady stream of research grants, perhaps along with industry-paid speaking fees and consulting contracts.

Of course, none of this means that industry-funded scientists conduct fraudulent research or that their conclusions are necessarily invalid. Industry-funded studies are frequently published in peer-reviewed journals and corroborated by nonindustry- or government-funded studies. But researchers' financial ties to sponsors do create a potential for bias that needs to be taken into account.

Whether or not industry provides funding or attempts to influence studies, food manufacturers commonly hire public relations firms to spread the word about research that promotes their commercial interests. The job of these PR firms is to stir up as much media attention as possible, which can entail spinning the facts to make research findings seem more important and definitive than they actually are. If PR professionals told the full truth, we might expect to see something like this: "A small study has found that food X temporarily raises blood levels of a substance that may have something to do with cancer, but it's unclear what, if any, relevance this has to human health." That would go nowhere in attracting publicity, of course, so instead the pitch becomes, "Food X may prevent cancer!" It's far sexier and much more likely to grab the attention of journalists.

A common PR technique in press releases is to omit or bury certain crucial details—for example, that the study was conducted on lab animals, or included only a small number of subjects, or was very short-term, or didn't include a control group. PR announcements may also present impressive-sounding relative benefits without providing absolute numbers that put the findings in context. In addition, press packages sometimes include strongly worded quotes from the researchers that aren't justified by the study's findings. Despite scientists' customary caution in interpreting research, such overstatement may occur when they succumb to pressure from industry and public relations professionals to simplify their findings and put them in layman's terms. It may also result from the recognition that strong statements can generate more media publicity, possibly raising researchers' prominence, bringing in more funding, and advancing their careers.

In some cases, other entities seeking publicity, such as the scientific journal in which the study was published, the health association sponsoring the meeting where it was presented, or the university with which the researcher is affiliated, may issue their own press announcements touting the research. Though they aren't trying to sell a food, they share industry's goal of generating as much media coverage as possible. And to that end, they too may exaggerate and present facts selectively.

Recognizing the public's strong interest in stories about food and health, reporters and editors typically pay attention when such news crosses their desks. After all, they're in the business of attracting an audience, and stories about foods with miraculous life-saving powers are sure to do the trick. Journalists typically learn of superfood research from press releases and may rely on them heavily—or even exclusively—in putting together their reports. Whether because of naïveté, laziness, tight deadlines, or some combination of these, reporters too often accept spinmeisters' version of the truth without question, sometimes passing along facts almost exactly as presented in news releases.

The television version of this practice is to use scripts, footage, and "sound bites" supplied by PR professionals. These ready-to-use news reports, known as video news releases, or VNRs, are essentially propaganda disguised as news. VNRs have become the subject of great controversy and criticism in recent years, but they continue to be widely used by stations of all sizes, according to a study by the Center for Media and Democracy. It found that local news shows typically present VNRs as their own journalism and rarely verify the information contained in the stories or add anything to them.

Whether the source is a VNR or a press release, media stories about superfoods don't always disclose who funded the research. And when they do, this information may appear only in a brief mention buried within the report or tacked on at the end. Further, press announcements sometimes include quotes (or sound bites) from "independent" experts who are in fact paid by industry. Their ties to industry often aren't revealed to journalists, who end up using the quotes without proper disclosure.

This relationship among industry, researchers, public relations firms, and journalists works to the advantage of all parties involved. Researchers get funding and attention. Public relations firms get lucrative contracts. The media get attention-grabbing stories handed to them. And industry gets its message out. The big loser, though, is the public, which gets duped into believing that specific foods will magically keep illness away. Not only may people develop a false sense of security, reassured that they're protecting themselves from disease, but they may also end up consuming more calories than they need (and thereby negatively affecting their health) as they stuff themselves with supposedly life-saving foods.

NUTTY CLAIMS

The marketing of walnuts serves as just one illustration of how the industry/PR/media spin machine operates. A decent body of research links eating nuts of all types with a lower risk of heart disease, and it's reasonable to conclude that they can be part of a healthful diet when consumed in moderation. But growers of walnuts, in an attempt to distinguish their products from their nutty brothers, have gone a step further, aggressively pushing walnuts as "the 21st Century 'Super Food'" and an "essential food for health" that is "packed with nutrients that positively affect the body on a multitude of levels."

One such nutrient is alpha-linolenic acid (ALA), an omega-3 fat that the body converts in small amounts into the heart-healthy forms known as DHA and EPA, which are found in fish. ALA is present in not only walnuts but also soybeans and soybean oil, canola oil, and leafy green vegetables. Flaxseed contains the highest levels. A study of 20 men and three women, funded by the California Walnut Commission and published in the *Journal of Nutrition*, tested short-term physiological effects of a diet relatively high in ALA. After six weeks on this diet, which included walnuts, walnut oil, and flaxseed oil, subjects experienced a drop in C-reactive protein, a measure of inflammation that may be associated with heart disease. Other inflammatory markers, known as adhesion molecules, also decreased, as did cholesterol levels.

To publicize the findings, the California Walnut Commission issued a press announcement with the bold headline: "New Proof: Walnuts Show Multiple New Heart Health Benefits." Never mind that a six-week study with only 23 subjects can't really provide "proof" of much of anything. Attributing the apparent benefits entirely to walnuts, the release did not mention that the diet high in ALA also included flaxseed oil. Nor did it disclose that the Walnut Commission had funded the study.

What it did include was an assertion that the fats in walnuts are just as beneficial as those in fish. This was misleading, however, because the study had not compared the effects of walnuts directly to those of fish. And the benefits of omega-3 fats in fish are far better documented than those of ALA found in plant sources such as walnuts. What's more, some evidence hints (though certainly doesn't prove) that higher intakes of ALA may increase the risk of advanced prostate cancer. But none of this was made clear in most news reports about the research, which tended to parrot the walnut industry's characterization of walnuts as an alternative to fish:

> "By now, you've likely heard that a diet rich in certain types of fish helps ward off heart attacks and strokes. But if you can't stand the thought of eating fish, take heart—and try walnuts instead."
>
> (WebMD)

> "Experts say a one-ounce serving of walnuts has more than 2.5 grams of omega-3s, somewhat more than the average 1.46 grams in 3 ounces of Atlantic-farmed salmon."
>
> (*Health* magazine)

"High fish consumption decreases the risk of heart attacks because of omega-3 fatty acids. . . . The Penn State study shows that plant sources of the omega-3s do the same thing. The study is valuable because of health concerns about eating fish like salmon frequently."

(*Modesto Bee*)

Another ingredient the walnut industry is eager for us to know about is the hormone melatonin. In an industry-funded study published in the journal *Nutrition*, walnuts were analyzed for their levels of melatonin and then fed to 12 rats. A comparison group of rodents got their usual chow. The rats eating walnuts were found to have higher levels of melatonin and greater antioxidant activity in their blood.

Though melatonin's best-known use is for alleviating jet lag and insomnia, some researchers (including the study's lead author) have long touted it as an antioxidant that can prevent chronic disease and fight the effects of aging. While dozens of laboratory and animal studies have explored melatonin's antioxidant effects, and some research has linked higher melatonin levels in people with lower disease rates, there are no long-term human trials proving that taking the hormone in any form—whether through pills or plant sources such as walnuts—actually prevents disease.

But that didn't stop walnut industry spinners from presenting melatonin's disease-fighting ability as an established fact. And they took an additional leap in scientific logic with this overblown assertion in a press release headline: "New Study Shows Melatonin in Walnuts Protective against Cancer and Heart Disease." Of course, the study had found no such thing—not even in rats. Given the exaggeration, it's not surprising that the release also neglected to mention that the study was conducted on lab animals or that it was funded by the walnut industry.

A video news release from the walnut industry was even more misleading because of scientifically baseless sound bites from the study's lead author, Russel Reiter of the University of Texas Health Science Center in San Antonio. Among them:

"Consuming walnuts would be expected to either prevent or delay or modify the incidence of cancer, the progression of neurodegenerative diseases, and the frequency of cardiovascular degeneration."

"I don't think there's any doubt that consuming walnuts on a regular basis—because of their nutritional ingredients—would, in fact, improve the quality of life for individuals as they age."

"Walnuts are an exceptionally good food. When you include them in your diet, you can be expected to improve your general health. To not include them is foolhardy."

Reiter, who received $50,000 from the California Walnut Commission to conduct the study, says that no one tried to influence his comments and that he stands by them. Nevertheless, he acknowledges, "You don't want to bite the hand that feeds you."

Certainly, walnuts aren't the only nuts being marketed this way. Producers of almonds, pecans, and peanuts (which technically aren't nuts but legumes) also use science and the media to promote the supposedly unique health-promoting properties of their particular nuts. The truth is that while nuts differ in their levels of various ingredients, no nut has been proven superior to others. Nor is any nut a miracle food. A sensible approach, then, is to eat a variety of nuts you enjoy, especially as a replacement for sugary snacks or animal fats. But because they're relatively high in calories, don't go nuts and eat the whole can in one sitting.

SWEET DREAMS

If there were prizes for superfoods, the "most improved" award would have to go to chocolate. Though it has long been regarded as a guilty pleasure full of fat and empty calories, numerous studies have now proven chocolate to be a health food that can reduce the risk of heart disease. At least that's the message being marketed by the chocolate industry through the news media. As is the case with other superfoods, however, the truth is far more complicated.

Cocoa, a main ingredient in chocolate, is high in antioxidants known as flavanols, which are also found in red wine, tea, and certain fruits. (In some discussions of chocolate, you might see the term "flavonoids," which is a broader category of compounds that includes flavanols.) The processing of chocolate can substantially reduce flavanol levels, leaving many popular chocolates nearly devoid of the compounds. In general, dark chocolate is richer in flavanols than milk chocolate, and much of the research has focused on the dark variety.

Some epidemiological studies have found an association between high flavanol intake (typically from sources other than chocolate) and lower rates of heart attacks and heart disease deaths, while other studies have found no relationship. As for chocolate-specific research, laboratory studies and small, short-term human experiments suggest that cocoa may positively affect the cardiovascular system by improving blood vessel function, lowering blood pressure and cholesterol, and making blood less likely to clot. But it's not known whether the effects are long-lasting or whether they lead to lower rates of heart disease and strokes.

For years, the giant candy maker Mars Inc. has been developing its own high-flavanol dark chocolate and has funded university-based research on chocolate's health effects, using the study findings to promote its products and to create a buzz in the media about the benefits of chocolate. A steady stream of news reports about the research has helped generate the impression that there's a growing mountain of definitive evidence, when, in fact, most of the studies are small and preliminary.

To get its message across, Mars is also quick to promote findings from research it hasn't funded. One example is a study in the journal *Hypertension*, a publication of the American Heart Association, in which half the subjects ate flavanol-rich dark chocolate every day, while the other half got flavanol-free white chocolate. Then they switched and ate the other chocolate. The researchers found that blood pressure dropped after subjects ate dark chocolate but not white. Likewise, there were reductions in insulin resistance and LDL (bad) cholesterol among the dark chocolate eaters.

Mars jumped on the findings with a press release headlined "New Study Offers More Support for Potential Heart Health Benefits of Cocoa Flavanols." But the announcement failed to mention some key caveats: the research involved only 20 people, and the effects were measured for just 15 days, leaving unanswered questions about what, if any, long-term impact chocolate might have on people's health. Additionally, the subjects were fed special dark chocolate with much higher flavanol levels than those in typical chocolate products. And their daily dose, a 3.5-ounce bar, added a whopping 480 calories to their diets.

The American Heart Association issued its own press release, which was more balanced. Though it began with the prescriptive-sounding statement that "if you have high blood pressure, a daily bar-sized serving of flavonol-rich dark chocolate might lower your blood pressure and improve insulin resistance" (implying that you might want to try this), it went on to include cautionary comments from one of the researchers, who noted that "this study is not about eating more chocolate" and "the findings do not suggest that people with high blood pressure should eat lots of dark chocolate in lieu of other important blood pressure reduction methods." In the same vein, a newspaper article on the study included a quote from the same researcher stressing that the study was "not saying that chocolate is now a health food."

But in some cases, such efforts to put the findings into perspective were overshadowed or even directly contradicted by headlines and lead paragraphs (which are all that many people read). For example, a report from Knight Ridder News Service, headlined "A Sweet Treatment for High Blood Pressure," began this way: "For those with hypertension, a daily dose of dark chocolate may be just what the doctor ordered." Readers had to get to the last paragraph for the caveats that "the findings do not mean people should gorge on dark chocolate" and that "more study is needed."

At least there were *some* caveats. Local television reports on the research often failed to include any at all, as these examples indicate:

> "It's another excuse to indulge your sweet tooth. A small study found high blood pressure patients who ate three and a half ounces of dark chocolate showed a drop in blood pressure. They also showed an improvement in insulin sensitivity. The cocoa contains natural chemicals called flavonoids that are good for your body."
>
> (KSDK, St. Louis)

> "If you needed another reason to eat more chocolate, the American Heart Association is giving you one more. According to a new study in *Hypertension*, some dark chocolate may be good for high blood pressure."
>
> (WJW, Cleveland)

"There is more conclusive evidence chocolate is good for you. Researchers found dark chocolate can lower blood pressure. The study joins a growing body of research that shows compounds in chocolate called flavonoids can help the blood vessels work."

(KRCG, Jefferson City, Missouri)

"A great excuse to eat some chocolate, according to a study in the journal of the American Heart Association. Some forms of dark chocolate may be good for people with high blood pressure. Researchers found that flavonoids in dark chocolate reduced blood pressure significantly and also produced a drop in bad cholesterol."

(KVUE, Austin)

The American Heart Association does not encourage people to eat more chocolate. But by publicizing the findings and thereby making them seem to be a big deal, the AHA further contributed to the Mars-led media hype and gave the impression (as evidenced by some of the television coverage) that it endorsed chocolate as medicine. The organization's purpose in issuing a press release was presumably to draw attention to its journal, but its action ended up advancing the interests of chocolate manufacturers.

If chocolate makers, researchers, and the media were being completely truthful, here's what they'd tell us: While preliminary research suggests that relatively large amounts of dark chocolate might have short-term, positive effects on the cardiovascular system, it's unknown whether there are any long-term benefits, which is what matters. It's certainly okay to treat yourself to chocolate now and then, and if you want to hedge your bets and go with dark chocolate, fine. But because it's high in calories, don't overdo it. And remember that whether dark or light, chocolate is, after all, candy—not medicine.

DAIRY DECEPTION

Of all the groups seeking superfood status for their products, none has been more aggressive than the dairy industry. Its message: milk isn't just wholesome and nutritious, as several generations of schoolchildren have been taught to believe, but can actually ward off disease. As part of the dairy industry's famous "Got Milk?" ad campaign, celebrities ranging from Leann Rimes to Garfield the cat have been enlisted to sport milk mustaches and instruct us that the beverage guards against osteoporosis and the bone fractures that can result from the condition.

The industry also spreads the word through a steady stream of press announcements about research on milk and bone health, which the media then dutifully relay to the public. In some cases, those studies are conducted by industry-funded scientists and published in industry-supported sections of journals. But typically such details aren't included in the press releases.

For example, one release—issued, ironically, on April Fool's Day— announced that a "definitive new research review" had concluded that "a diet devoid of dairy products could lead to bone fractures." What the announcement didn't reveal was that the researcher, Dr. Robert Heaney of Creighton University, was a recipient of dairy industry funding and a leading proponent of dairy's benefits. Nor was it disclosed that this review, along with other laudatory studies about dairy, had appeared in a special supplement to the *Journal of the American College of Nutrition* sponsored by the International Dairy Federation. One of the two guest editors of the supplement, who, in the words of the journal, "are responsible for the scientific merit of the articles," was an official of the National Dairy Council. The incestuousness of it all certainly called into question the independence and credibility of the research. But from a marketing perspective, that didn't matter; it was just another opportunity, created by the industry, to reinforce the notion that there's definitive proof of the bone-building benefits of milk and that we all need to drink more of it.

It's certainly true that calcium is necessary for strong bones and that milk and other dairy products are rich sources of calcium. But despite what the industry would have us believe, the evidence is mixed regarding milk's effect on bones, with some research finding that high dairy consumption does not reduce the risk of fractures. One review of the science determined that "most studies of dairy food intake and bone health provided inconclusive results."

It's also worth noting that in countries such as China and Japan, where consumption of dairy products is low, rates of fractures are also relatively low. What this suggests is that bone health is determined by more than how much milk we drink; it's a function of, among other things, genetics, physical activity, body size, hormone levels, animal protein (too much may leach calcium from bones), vitamin D intake, and sun exposure (which causes the skin to make vitamin D). What's more, calcium can also come from non-dairy sources, such as dark green leafy vegetables, canned salmon, and dried beans and peas as well as fortified products. Though these foods typically contain less calcium than dairy products do, it's quite possible to get adequate amounts of the mineral—and to protect your bones—through means other than milk. The dairy industry, of course, prefers that we swallow its overzealous endorsement of milk as something everyone needs for strong bones.

If fear of disintegrating bones isn't reason enough to persuade you to get your daily dairy fix, the industry has added another—and even more controversial—claim: that milk and other dairy products promote weight loss. In a massive marketing effort that included celebrity milk mustache ads, community events, and weight loss contests with cash prizes, the dairy industry hawked the idea that three daily servings of dairy can help dieters lose more weight and burn more fat.

A key part of this campaign, according to an industry presentation, was "selling the science," because people "want facts and proof." But there was little solid science to sell—a fact that eventually forced the dairy industry to discontinue the effort. The bulk of the "proof" consisted of a few small, short-term human experiments conducted by Michael Zemel, an industry-funded researcher with the University of Tennessee, who zealously promotes the dairy–weight loss connection.

Zemel has profited nicely from this preliminary work by patenting the claim that high-calcium diets can treat or prevent obesity and selling exclusive licensing rights to the dairy industry and General Mills. He has also written a book whose "proven premise" is "eat more calcium-rich foods, lose more weight." The author's "revolutionary diet discovery," according to the book, will "speed up your metabolism" and "work wonders for your individual weight loss needs."

Similar studies by other investigators have found no evidence that dairy promotes weight loss. And even Zemel has acknowledged that his findings apply only to overweight people whose diets are low in calcium to begin with. But the dairy industry's ads, which typically showed people who weren't overweight, implied that everyone could lose weight on a dairy diet.

The industry's announcements to the press often conveyed the same misleading message, as did the resulting news reports. Some of the headlines and story leads sounded as though they were written by the industry itself:

DAIRY CALCIUM MAY AID WEIGHT LOSS AND BURN FAT
"Got milk? If you want to lose weight, perhaps you should have some."

([Florida] *Sun-Sentinel*)

BEHOLD THE POWER OF DAIRY
"It's not just for strong bones and healthy muscles; milk does your metabolism good."

([Mississippi] *Sun Herald*)

15 THINGS YOU NEED TO KNOW ABOUT MILK
"Milk is a natural weight-loss food. . . . By keeping calcium intake high and drinking plenty of milk, you can more than double the speed at which you lose weight. The place it comes off first? Your middle!"

(*Men's Fitness* magazine)

A video news release from the dairy industry resulted in similar messages on many TV news programs. Describing the "dramatic findings" from one of Zemel's industry-funded studies (and never mentioning who had paid for it), the VNR featured the researcher, who said the study showed "if you're cutting calories, you can make that effort about twice as effective" with three daily servings of dairy. In another sound bite, a registered dietician—who just happened to work for the National Dairy Council—hailed the findings as "great nutrition news because people enjoy eating dairy foods." Later, she advised viewers that all it takes is including milk in your morning cereal, cheese on your sandwich at lunch, and yogurt as your afternoon snack. And voilà, the video implied, you'll be slim in time for swimsuit season. Of course, the report did not include any experts questioning the research or the industry's claims. Though one news director in Cincinnati admitted that his station had erred by showing this piece of propaganda, many others in cities ranging from Boston to Sacramento used the footage, apparently without such qualms.

Whether your purpose is to lose weight or build bones, the advice to eat more dairy may seem fairly innocuous. After all, what harm can come from simply drinking more milk? For starters, it can lead to nausea, cramps, and diarrhea in many people because they lack the enzyme necessary to digest lactose, the sugar in milk. Further, 2 percent and whole milk are relatively high in saturated fat, the type associated with an increased risk of heart disease. Additionally, some studies—though not all—have linked higher milk and dairy consumption with an increased risk of prostate and ovarian cancer. This research doesn't prove that milk causes cancer, nor does it warrant steering clear of dairy. But it raises at least the possibility of drawbacks— something to keep in mind before swallowing the industry's promises that loading up on dairy will make us healthier. While milk and other dairy products certainly can be part of a healthful diet, they aren't necessary for good health.

LABEL CLAIMS

Food manufacturers have been emboldened to step up their health claims in part because of more permissive FDA rules about what's allowed on labels. Until recently, the agency gave its official blessing to claims only when they were backed up by "significant scientific agreement" or an authoritative statement from a federal scientific body like the National Academy of Sciences. For example, the FDA has allowed claims that low-fat diets rich in fruits and vegetables may reduce the risk of certain cancers; foods high in potassium and low in sodium may decrease the risk of high blood pressure and stroke; and diets rich in whole grains and low in fat may reduce the risk of heart disease and certain cancers.

But now the FDA, yielding to pressure from the food industry, also permits "qualified" health claims—those for which we have only limited evidence. The first group to get the green light was the walnut industry, which is allowed to state on labels that "supportive but not conclusive research shows that eating 1.5 ounces per day of walnuts, as part of a low saturated fat and low cholesterol diet and not resulting in increased caloric intake, may reduce the risk of coronary heart disease." Sellers of tomatoes and tomato sauce can make similarly equivocal claims that "very limited and preliminary scientific research suggests" that these foods may reduce the risk of prostate cancer. An FDA study found that consumers perceive claims like these to be *more* believable than other approved claims—just the opposite of what was intended.

Under food labeling laws, food manufacturers can also make certain types of claims without having to prove anything at all to the FDA. Known as "structure/function" claims, these describe how some food or nutrient affects normal functioning or well-being—for example, it "helps maintain healthy cholesterol levels" or "helps promote healthy blood pressure." The trick is that the claims don't explicitly say the food treats or prevents disease (for example, "lowers cholesterol"), which is forbidden without FDA approval. This subtle—and silly—distinction is lost on most of us, of course, and we simply infer that the product is good for us. Even though the FDA often requires structure/function claims to be accompanied by the disclaimer that "these statements have not been evaluated by the Food and Drug Administration," it's easy to overlook. The upshot is that food manufacturers can get away with making misleading claims under this labeling loophole as long as they're careful and clever with their wording.

Because claims on labels don't always convey the full truth and can be hard to decipher, they're not much help in countering industry spin and media hype about superfoods. So we're on our own to make sense of what we hear. When you encounter news about a particular food's amazing power to protect your health, you should begin by assuming that the report is *not* credible and conclude otherwise only if you get satisfactory answers to key questions about the research (listed in chapter 1).

Based on these criteria, superfood news is likely to come up short in most cases. So instead of worrying about whether to eat one specific food or another, stay focused on the big picture, incorporating a variety of foods from a few broad categories:

– Fruits and vegetables (the more colors, the better)

– Whole grains (including breads, cereals, and brown rice)

– Nuts and beans

– Fish (especially fatty fish such as salmon, tuna, and mackerel)

Decades of research suggest that a diet rich in foods from these categories—and relatively low in junk food, refined carbohydrates (such as white bread and sugary cereals), and red and processed meats—is the one most likely to confer health benefits. As alluring as it may be that magical-sounding food constituents—whether flavanols, retinols, isoflavones, lycopene, or anything else—represent the secret to health and longevity, what really matter are our overall eating and lifestyle patterns. No single food, regardless of its level of such ingredients, can make up for an otherwise unhealthful diet. The good news, though, is that focusing on broad categories rather than specific foods and their ingredients makes eating far easier and more enjoyable. A mixed fruit salad seems a lot more appetizing, after all, than a cup of antioxidants.

TRUSTWORTHY SOURCES OF INFORMATION

Nutrition Action Healthletter (www.cspinet.org) from the consumer watchdog group Center for Science in the Public Interest. Though derided by some as the "food police," CSPI publishes a highly practical and lively newsletter that objectively weighs the science and puts confusing information in context.

Tufts Health and Nutrition Letter (www.healthletter.tufts.edu). Another terrific publication with useful evidence-based information.

Berkeley Wellness Letter (www.wellnessletter.com). This newsletter offers a balanced, bottom-line approach to not only nutrition but also a host of wellness issues.

(Note: None of the three newsletters listed above accepts advertising.)

The Nutrition Source, Harvard School of Public Health (www.hsph .harvard.edu/nutritionsource). This informative, balanced Web site for consumers is the creation of prominent Harvard researchers whose work, which includes several large cohort studies, has revealed much of what we know about food and health.

What to Eat, by Marion Nestle (New York: North Point Press, 2006). Nestle, one of the nation's foremost nutrition experts and a frequent critic of the food industry, provides an informative aisle-by-aisle guide to supermarket shopping.

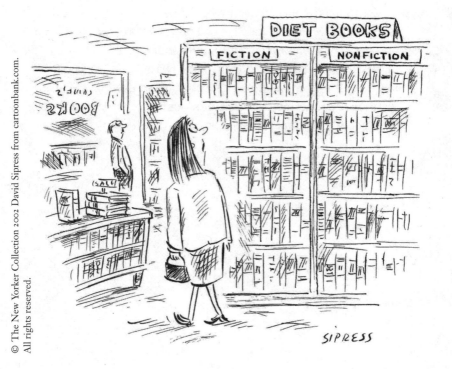

© The New Yorker Collection 2002 David Sipress from cartoonbank.com.
All rights reserved.

CHAPTER THREE: DIET BOOKS
DON'T EAT THAT!

What killed the famous diet doctor? No, I'm not referring to the famous case of the Scarsdale Diet doctor, Herman Tarnower, who was murdered by his lover. Nor is this a plot from an Agatha Christie novel or an episode of a TV detective show. It's a real-life mystery that has never been solved and remains a matter of intense speculation. The doctor is Robert Atkins, the force behind one of the most popular weight loss plans of all time. Critics have long charged that his diet, which shuns carbohydrates in favor of fat-laden foods, increases the risk of heart disease. Atkins claimed just the opposite, declaring through his doctor that he had an "extraordinarily healthy cardiovascular system" thanks to his diet.

In 2003, Atkins died at age 72, after suffering head injuries from a fall. That much is known. But controversy abounds over what caused the fall—a slippery sidewalk, as his family says, or a massive heart attack or stroke, as some groups opposed to his diet allege. (A year earlier, Atkins had suffered cardiac arrest, which he said stemmed from a heart infection and was "in no way related to diet.") Then there's the question of Atkins's weight when he died. The New York City medical examiner's report put it at 258 pounds, which at his height of 6 feet would have made Atkins obese. His widow says he weighed 195 pounds when he was admitted to the hospital but gained 60 pounds from fluid retention during the eight days that he lay in a coma.

Though his critics have pressed for more information, they are unlikely to ever receive definitive answers, at least publicly. There was no autopsy, and Atkins's widow won't release his medical records, calling her husband's medical history "private and of no concern or relevance to the media or general public." So we're left to guess whether the doctor's own diet may have done him in.

Of course, even if Atkins was obese and suffering from heart disease, his individual experience doesn't prove or disprove anything about his diet. Nevertheless, the Atkins mystery serves as a metaphor for the uncertainties surrounding popular weight loss regimens, especially those like the Atkins plan that instruct us to avoid specific foods. Is eschewing pineapples, potatoes, steaks, or sweets really the secret to staying slim, as various diets assure us? And, as we frequently hear, will shedding pounds make us healthier and extend our lives? The evidence for these assertions is surprisingly thin. Just as we lack definitive information about Dr. Atkins's weight and health, it's not always clear how dieting affects our own weight and health. What research *does* clearly suggest is that we'd be better off forgetting about diet plans and focusing instead on fitness and lifestyle.

WEIGHT LOSS CLAIMS

Like superfood proponents, who identify dietary heroes that supposedly keep us healthy, many popular diet plans point to villains that allegedly make us fat. Low-carb diets such as Atkins and South Beach, for example, initially ban fruit, bread, potatoes, pasta, carrots, and corn, among other things, and urge people to forswear some foods for good. The Suzanne Somers diet, which dubs sugar "the body's greatest enemy," condemns many of the same foods, plus pumpkin, parsnips, butternut squash, and skim milk. The Ornish diet gives a thumbs-down to meats, vegetable oils, nuts, seeds, avocados, and egg yolks. And under the Eat Right 4 Your Type diet, you're supposed to stay away from dairy and wheat products if you have type O blood; meat if you have type A; chicken, peanuts, and potatoes if you have type B; and turkey and bananas if you have type AB. Got that?

With a combined total of tens of millions of copies in print, these and other diet books regularly top best-seller lists. Not coincidentally, many promise dramatic results: you can "lose every ounce of excess weight that you need to," "shed pounds for good," "lose weight for life," and "reprogram your metabolism," while "eating more food than you ever have in your life." The diets, based on "breakthrough research," are touted as "scientifically proven to help you lose weight" and even "foolproof" for achieving "fast and healthy weight loss." By following these plans, you can have a "trimmer waist, better health in just ten days" and "join the ranks of the fit and fabulous."

The books' authors, flogging their diets in media interviews, often resort to rhetoric that's just as overblown. For example, Robert Atkins, appearing on CNN, declared that the evidence was "overwhelming" that his diet leads to greater fat loss than others. "There's no question," he asserted, that it lets you "eat unlimited quantities and still lose weight." Similarly, Dr. Arthur Agatston, interviewed on *Dateline NBC* about his South Beach diet, said that he was "just absolutely amazed by the results with my patients," because his diet allows them to "lose weight, have wonderful blood chemistry, and not be hungry, and eat very well."

Some of the most outlandish statements have come from Suzanne Somers (of *Three's Company* and Thighmaster fame), author of a series of blockbuster diet books. On the *Today Show*, she boasted, "I've had people lose 100, 150, 200, 250 pounds. Incredible." ("Incredible" indeed, given that there are only anecdotes and no published research to back up such assertions.) Discussing one of her recipes—a soufflé pancake made of cream cheese and eggs—during another appearance on *Today*, Somers claimed that "you can't gain weight because there's no sugar." And on CNN, she made a similarly science-defying promise: "By eliminating sugar and not eating fat and carbohydrate together, you won't have cellulite. And the cellulite you have will eventually melt away."

Sensational claims like these don't hold up when subjected to rigorous, independent research. In a randomized trial published in the *Journal of the American Medical Association (JAMA)*, for example, 160 overweight or obese participants were assigned to one of four diets: Atkins, Ornish, Weight Watchers, or the Zone. After one year, participants on the Atkins

diet lost, on average, just about 5 pounds. Those on the other diets lost a
pound or two more, though the differences weren't statistically significant. A big problem, especially for Atkins and Ornish dieters, was adherence. Few got their carb or fat intake down to the recommended levels,
and about half of the subjects on these plans threw in the towel before the
study was over.

Another diet-comparison trial published in *JAMA* gave a slight edge to
Atkins but, like the other study, found average weight loss for all diets to
be modest and adherence rates low. Other randomized studies report that
in the short term (up to six months), low-carb diets like Atkins result in
greater weight loss than conventional diets that cut calories and fat. But
after a year, low-carb's apparent advantages disappear, with both ap-
proaches leading to roughly equal and relatively small weight changes on
average.

Studies of low-fat diets have produced equally unimpressive results. For
example, a review of research by the highly respected Cochrane Collaboration concluded that fat-restricted diets were no more effective than calorie-
restricted diets, with subjects, on average, losing about 5 pounds after 12
months and returning to their original weight after 18 months. Likewise,
the Women's Health Initiative study, which randomly assigned subjects to
either a low-fat or a control diet, found that after seven and a half years,
average weights for the two groups were about the same.

If you want further evidence that banishing bananas, bologna, or other
bad guys isn't a silver bullet for shedding pounds, consider what happened
in the 1980s and 1990s: millions of Americans embraced the notion, disseminated by diet peddlers, the media, and some weight loss experts, that
eating fat is what makes us fat. In a sign of just how deeply ingrained the
idea became, the writers of the hit TV sitcom *Seinfeld* built an entire
episode around it. Titled "The Non-Fat Yogurt," the 1993 episode has the
characters marveling over the taste of one store's nonfat yogurt, with Jerry's
overweight nemesis, Newman, enthusiastically declaring, "I've been waiting
for something like this my whole life!" But when Jerry and Elaine both
learn they've inexplicably put on weight, they suspect the yogurt must contain fat. Sending it to a lab to be tested, they confirm that to be the case and

expose the fraud. Newman, furious at Jerry for spoiling his pleasure, says, "I will get even with you for this. You can count on it."

Like Jerry, Elaine, and Newman, many of us wrongly assumed that foods without fat were nonfattening. Steering clear of fat-containing products from soup to nuts, we loaded up instead on carbohydrates like bread and pasta. The food industry, eager to capitalize on our anti-fat fetish, flooded the market with low- and no-fat cookies, crackers, chips, and ice cream. It was okay to overindulge in such foods, we concluded, heedless of the fact that they often contain roughly as many calories as (and more sugar than) their higher-fat counterparts.

We all know what happened: the low-fat strategy, at least as followed by most people, failed. While we consumed less fat as a percentage of calories, our total calorie intake went up, and so did our weight. Along came Dr. Atkins—actually, he'd been around for decades peddling his diet—with a diagnosis: it was the carbs that were making us fat. He and like-minded diet promoters argued that carbs cause blood sugar to rise rapidly, triggering a surge of insulin that then makes blood sugar levels plummet, leading to hunger and cravings for more carbs.

Though carbs may be a contributing factor, they have never been proven to be the main reason for weight gain, as the champions of low-carb diets assert. Nevertheless, many people have swallowed this theory as gospel, forsaking beans for bacon and carrots for cheese. Instead of recognizing that calories, physical activity, and genetics are what matter when it comes to weight, we've simply fallen for another fad, a variation on the unproven theme that it's all about what foods we exclude. And, once again, the food industry is indulging us in our fantasy, churning out low-carb snacks, desserts, and other foods that many wrongly believe can be eaten to excess with impunity.

If you resist such temptations, a diet that bans particular foods can indeed help you lose weight in the short term. The real issue, though, is whether it's sustainable over the long run and allows you to keep the weight off. That's where the vast majority of dieters get tripped up, with about 95 percent eventually regaining lost weight. One reason is that most diets, especially those that cut out particular foods, leave us feeling deprived, and we fall back on our old eating habits.

HEALTH CLAIMS

Even if "don't eat that" diets fail to keep weight off long-term, we assume that they at least benefit our health and well-being. That's certainly the promise of many popular plans, as articulated by their proponents:

> "You will substantially increase your odds of living long and well—meaning you will maintain your health and vitality as you age. . . . I'm not exaggerating when I say that this diet, as a fringe benefit, can save your life."
>
> (Dr. Arthur Agatston)

> "You will achieve good health. The change is amazing. . . . You become less tired and more energetic, not merely because of weight loss but because the physical consequences of a truly dysfunctional blood sugar and insulin metabolism are reversed."
>
> (Dr. Robert Atkins)

> "Most people find they feel so much better so quickly that it reframes the reasons for changing diet from fear of dying to joy of living. You have more energy because . . . your brain really does get more blood flow. That's been shown. We have shown in our studies that the heart gets more blood flow within weeks, and scientifically it has been shown that sexual organs get more blood flow, too."
>
> (Dr. Dean Ornish)

Once again, however, the science doesn't fully support the diet pushers' assertions. It is true, according to several studies, that low-carb diets can have a beneficial effect on HDL (good) cholesterol and blood fats called triglycerides, at least in the short run. Restricting carbs can also help improve responsiveness to insulin in those whose bodies are resistant to it. But whether these improvements persist long-term—and therefore lead to a lower risk of disease—is unknown.

Low-carb diets that severely restrict fruits, vegetables, and whole grains can cause constipation, headaches, and fatigue. More seriously, there's also the possibility (though it's never been proven) that they may put us at greater risk of cancer and heart disease by leaving us deficient in certain nutrients. Dietary supplements, which some plans recommend to compensate for the cutback, generally don't pack the same nutritional punch as real food.

As for the notion that low-fat diets are good for us—something we've heard for decades—it's not that simple. A fat-restricted diet may indeed reduce LDL (bad) and total cholesterol, and research suggests that limiting saturated and trans fats may be beneficial. But reducing total fat doesn't appear to lower the risk of heart disease or certain cancers. And an extremely low-fat diet can have a negative impact on HDL (good) cholesterol and triglycerides and can exclude unsaturated fats such as those found in fish, nuts, and plant oils, which may help protect against cardiovascular disease.

Proponents of low-fat diets often point to a study, led by Dr. Dean Ornish and published in *JAMA*, reporting that heart patients who ate a vegetarian diet that contained only 10 percent fat actually experienced a reversal of their condition. But the research included fewer than 50 subjects and also involved other lifestyle changes such as exercise, smoking cessation, and stress management training, making it hard to isolate the exact effects of diet.

The truth is that simply minimizing or eliminating carbohydrates or fats doesn't necessarily make a diet more healthful. It depends on the types (refined or unrefined carbs, saturated or unsaturated fats) as well as what you replace those foods with. If you stop eating white bread, you may be helping your health if you choose the whole-wheat variety instead, but not if you forgo the bread for fatty meats. Likewise, cutting out potato chips as a snack is an improvement if you switch to nuts or fruit, but not necessarily if you replace them with low-fat cookies.

WEIGHTY QUESTIONS

Beyond the issue of whether including or excluding particular foods is healthful, there's a more fundamental question: is shedding pounds, through whatever means, good for your health? This may seem like an odd thing to ask, given that so many diet promoters, doctors, and weight loss experts have drilled it into our heads that it's beneficial for overweight people to slim down. In fact, the research suggests that may not always be true.

It's known that in people who are obese (as defined by the body mass index, or BMI, scale, which takes height and weight into account), weight loss can help control or prevent high blood pressure and diabetes. It can also have positive effects on cholesterol, triglycerides, and C-reactive protein, an inflammatory marker linked to heart disease. Further, it may reduce the severity of sleep apnea, a potentially life-threatening condition. So you'd expect that losing weight would allow you to live longer. Though some research has found this to be the case, many studies suggest just the opposite: that people who lose weight actually have *higher* death rates than those whose weight has remained stable, even if they're overweight.

For example, in a cohort study of Harvard alumni, middle-aged men who either lost or gained weight had an increased likelihood of dying earlier, with the risk being highest in those who had lost 11 pounds or more. Similarly, an Israeli cohort study found that, compared to men whose weight remained stable, those who lost 11 pounds or more had a slightly higher mortality risk, both heart disease–related and overall. In a study conducted by the Centers for Disease Control and Prevention, which included men and women ages 45 to 74, overweight people who lost 15 percent or more of their body weight had higher death rates than those who lost less than 5 percent.

Such research has been criticized, however, for not adequately controlling for diseases or risk factors that might account for the higher death rates. Also, not all studies distinguished between intentional and unintentional weight loss. People who lose weight unintentionally may do so because of an undiagnosed illness. If this possibility isn't taken into consideration, studies that detect a higher mortality risk may wrongly conclude that weight loss is a *cause* of subjects' increased risk rather than the *result* of their impaired health status. To get accurate results, therefore, it's important that studies sort this out.

To that end, researchers analyzing data from the Finnish Twin Cohort study separated out the intentional from the unintentional weight losers and included only people who appeared to be free of illness. All were obese or overweight when the study began. Over an 18-year period, those who had lost weight on purpose were more likely to die than those whose weight had remained stable. The researchers concluded that deliberate weight loss in healthy, overweight people "may be hazardous in the long term."

Other cohort studies categorizing subjects according to their intention to lose weight and their health status have produced mixed results. In some cases, deliberate weight losers had higher death rates than those with no change in weight. In others (mainly when subjects had underlying health conditions such as diabetes), dieters' death rates were lower. And, in several instances, intentional weight loss had no effect on mortality one way or the other.

Though it's not clear why weight loss might increase mortality rates, a contributing factor may be that many dieters repeatedly lose and regain weight, a phenomenon known as yo-yo dieting. Some research has found that those with the greatest variability in their weight have the highest death rates. They also have a higher risk of diabetes, heart attacks, strokes, and hip fractures, among other things. Further, there's some evidence that yo-yo dieting may ultimately lead to even greater weight gain.

As a whole, the research suggests that dieting is not a risk-free endeavor and that in some cases the drawbacks may outweigh the benefits. The editors of the *New England Journal of Medicine* reached that conclusion in an editorial published on January 1, 1998. Under the headline "Losing Weight— An Ill-Fated New Year's Resolution," Drs. Jerome Kassirer and Marcia Angell wrote: "We simply do not know whether a person who loses 20 lb will thereby acquire the same reduced risk as a person who started out 20 lb lighter." Warning doctors to be cautious about urging all overweight patients to shed pounds, they said, "We should remember that the cure for obesity may be worse than the condition."

Though we have few definitive answers when it comes to weight loss, a careful review of the evidence does suggest some conclusions that are worth weighing as you decide whether to go on a diet:

- BMI IS AN IMPERFECT BAROMETER. Body mass index, the standard yardstick
for determining who needs to lose weight, is calculated by multiplying
weight in pounds by 703, dividing by height in inches, then dividing by
height again. A reading of 18.5 to 24.9 indicates that your weight is
normal; 25 to 29.9 means that you're overweight; and 30 and over
earns you the label of obese. According to this scale, the average
American woman, who's 5 feet 4 inches tall and weighs 164 pounds, is
overweight. So is the average American man, with a BMI of about 28.
Remarkably, two-thirds of American adults fall into the overweight or
obese range on the BMI scale, a group that includes George Clooney,
Cal Ripken, and Governor Arnold Schwarzenegger. The problem is
that this relatively crude tool fails to take into account factors such as
age, gender, race, fitness level, muscle mass, or body fat. Nor does it
consider the location of excess weight.

Studies suggest that people with extra fat mainly around the waist
(an apple shape) may be at greater risk of various conditions than those
with fat concentrated elsewhere, such as the thighs, hips, and butt (pear
shape). Therefore, in assessing your weight, it's a good idea to look
beyond BMI and consider your waist size.

- HEALTH STATUS MATTERS. Dieting is most likely to be beneficial if you have
a condition or risk factor, such as diabetes, sleep apnea, osteoarthritis,
high blood pressure, or high cholesterol, that can be improved by losing weight. But if you're healthy and not severely overweight, it's wise
to first ask yourself some hard questions: Am I willing to accept unknown, and possibly adverse, health consequences in order to try to
improve my appearance? Is the effort worth it, knowing that most
diets don't work very well and that I'm likely to eventually regain any
lost weight? Am I prepared to deal with the negative impact that failed
dieting could have on my emotional well-being?

- NEITHER DOOMSAYERS NOR DENIERS TELL THE FULL TRUTH. Many diet promoters, as well as some prominent obesity researchers and public health
officials, sound dire warnings about being overweight or obese, equat-
ing its effects with those of smoking. Some claim that excess pounds
are killing 400,000 Americans a year—an implausibly high figure con-

tradicted by CDC research putting the death toll at a fraction of that number—and even blame weight issues for everything from suicides to global warming. Lumping overweight and obesity together, they exaggerate what's known about the harms of excess weight and urge us to slim down or face deadly consequences. Suzanne Somers, for example, has exclaimed that "we are heading towards an obesity-related health crisis that economically will make AIDS look like the common cold," while another diet book author warns that "we are facing a public health disaster and potential economic collapse in the face of the accelerating obesity epidemic."

Many health promoters who spew out this hyperbole have a financial incentive to do so because they're promoting diets or consulting for companies that sell diet drugs and other weight loss remedies. Those who conduct research or head government health agencies also stand to benefit because the more urgent the problem seems, the more funding they're likely to get to address it.

On the other side are those who downplay or deny the problems associated with obesity. The most outspoken is the Center for Consumer Freedom, a nonprofit advocacy group formed with tobacco money and funded by the food and restaurant industries. The organization has run full-page newspaper ads featuring the word "hype" in bold red letters and warning that "Americans have been force-fed a steady diet of obesity myths by the 'food police,' trial lawyers, and even our own government." The center defends snacks, sodas, and junk food advertising to children, while hurling insults at those who advocate more healthful food options in schools or nutrition information in fast-food restaurants. Selectively citing evidence, this group and other deniers convey the misleading message, at least implicitly, that overeating is not a problem and that obesity poses little or no health threat.

The truth lies between these two extremes. While some studies have found higher weight to be associated with a somewhat greater risk of earlier death, others have concluded that people who are overweight are not at increased risk of dying from heart disease and cancer and actually have lower death rates overall than do those of normal weight. The inconsistencies are due in part to differences in study designs (such as including or excluding smokers) and in the populations studied. (African Americans and older people, for example, may have higher ideal BMIs than whites and younger people.) However, even studies that don't find serious hazards in being overweight show that obesity—especially extreme obesity—is associated with premature death. It also contributes to, and can worsen, a host of conditions ranging from asthma to cancer and increases the risk of disability. The growing number of overweight children is of special concern because many will grow up to be obese adults.

So while it's a distortion of science to claim that our expanding waistlines pose a deadly threat on the order of smoking, it's also an exaggeration to call the adverse effects of obesity a "myth." You shouldn't let the doomsayers' rhetoric scare you into trying the latest fad diet, nor should you let the deniers' assertions lull you into complacency over your eating habits, weight, and health.

THE ALTERNATIVE TO DIETING

So what are we supposed to do? Well, one thing is clear: what we're doing now is a dismal failure. With nearly half of U.S. adult women and one-third of men trying to lose weight, annual spending on weight loss products and services—including blockbuster diet books—is estimated to be $50 billion. Yet our waistlines continue to expand.

As the old saw goes, the definition of insanity is trying the same thing over and over and expecting different results. Next time you find yourself tempted to try yet another diet in the hope that this one, unlike all the others, will make you skinny, you might consider a different approach: focus less on weight and more on healthful living. Unlike many diet manuals, this method offers no guarantees that it will melt away pounds immediately, but it can reduce the harm associated with obesity, according to a substantial body of research. And, in the process, it can prevent weight gain—something research suggests is a good idea—and perhaps even lead to weight loss. This alternative approach involves three key components.

FITNESS

Many popular diets give short shrift to exercise, and some even boast that it's not required. For example, a full-page ad for a book on the South Beach diet has dubbed it a "no exercise-needed approach to weight loss." In fact, emphasizing dieting and downplaying exercise are exactly the opposite of what we should do. Research by Dr. Steven Blair, formerly of the Cooper Institute for Aerobics in Dallas and now with the University of South Carolina, has shown that it's possible to be both fit and fat and that regular exercise can offset the risks associated with obesity. He and his colleagues reported that men who were obese and fit actually had *lower* death rates than those who were thin and unfit. Other researchers, studying women, have concluded that fitness level is a more important contributor than weight to the risk of heart attacks, strokes, and death from cardiovascular disease.

Though some researchers don't agree that fitness trumps fatness when it comes to health, their studies show that obese people may at least lower their risk of heart disease and diabetes by being physically active. Regardless of which studies you choose, the consistent finding is that exercise, by itself, can help ameliorate—perhaps greatly—the health problems linked to obesity.

As Laura Fraser writes in *Losing It*, her exposé of the weight loss industry, many people who are overweight and sedentary don't start exercising because they're intimidated by ubiquitous images of "super-bodied athletes with high-performance gear." Believing that such images are far removed from their own reality, they don't even bother to try. In fact, you don't need special equipment to get fit, nor is it necessary to join a gym filled with hard-bodied people who make you feel self-conscious. Instead, activities such as walking, climbing stairs, doing housework, or gardening can do the trick. The key is just to get moving and to squeeze in a total of at least thirty minutes—whether continuously or in several short spurts—most days. If you can include activities you enjoy, you're more likely to stick with it.

Don't expect rapid or extreme weight loss from exercise. If you do, you're setting yourself up for disappointment and failure. The point of getting moving is to improve your health and to feel better physically and emotionally. If you shed pounds along the way, great, but it shouldn't be your main motivation.

HEALTHFUL FOOD CHOICES

Instead of trying to avoid specific foods, as many diets advise, you're better off concentrating on eating more healthfully. In addition to including more fruits, vegetables, whole grains, legumes, and fish, such a plan entails cutting back on less healthful foods like sodas, chips, cookies, crackers, and high-fat meats, cheeses, and ice cream. But it doesn't mean viewing these less desirable foods as poison and banishing them altogether, the way some diets blacklist specific foods. Instead, the idea is to make them occasional treats. If such foods are now part of your daily fare, try to cut back gradually. When you crave a candy bar, for example, try a piece of fruit every other time instead. That way, you won't feel deprived. Remember that your eating habits have developed over a lifetime, and you're most likely to succeed in changing them permanently—which is the goal—through slow and steady improvements. Diets that force you to immediately and drastically alter what you eat are doomed to fail because they expect too much, too soon.

Many healthful foods have the added advantage of being more filling. Foods such as fruits, vegetables, salads, and soups have lower "energy density"—meaning that they contain more water and therefore fewer calories per ounce—than, say, chips or pizza. Dr. Barbara Rolls and her colleagues at Pennsylvania State University report that by opting for less energy-dense foods, we can eat more and feel full on fewer calories.

In our supersized society, where giant orders of fries, massive muffins, and enormous entrees have become the norm, it's easy to overeat energy-dense foods that aren't especially healthful. As research by Professor Brian Wansink of Cornell University has shown, often we're oblivious to how much we're consuming. If a restaurant serves large portions, ask for a smaller amount or set aside part in a doggy bag before you start eating. If necessary, throw away some of those fries or part of that giant cookie so you won't be tempted to eat the whole serving. The idea is not to weigh food or count calories or deprive yourself, as many diets advise, but simply to pay closer attention to what—and how much—you're consuming.

MANAGING EXPECTATIONS ABOUT WEIGHT

The message conveyed by diet peddlers is that your weight is entirely within your control. If you choose a particular plan and follow it faithfully, they promise, you can have the body you want. For many women, that means resembling a super-thin supermodel or celebrity—the type of "ideal" body image that inundates us through television, movies, and magazine covers. In reality, weight is heavily influenced by genetics, and most women are not biologically programmed to look like Jennifer Aniston or Heidi Klum. No matter how much they diet, people who are prone to be heavier are unlikely to become skinny—and even if they do shrink substantially, their bodies eventually return to a higher weight. This doesn't mean we're completely powerless regarding our weight—just that there are limits to how much we can control. The failure to recognize this takes a huge psychological toll on women, with many developing self-esteem issues because they can't meet society's one-size-fits-all standard for slimness.

The notion that bodies come in all shapes and sizes underlies a strategy called "Health at Every Size," which encourages self-acceptance rather than the pursuit of an ideal weight. It also puts an emphasis on physical activity and healthful eating. Research by Dr. Linda Bacon and her colleagues at the University of California, Davis, suggests that this approach is more effective than dieting in producing long-term health improvements. In a randomized study of 78 obese women, half were instructed on the basics of dieting. The other half were told to forget about dieting and instead let the body's internal cues of hunger and fullness guide their eating. In addition, they participated in a support group focused on self-acceptance and self-esteem, while being taught how to choose healthful foods and overcome barriers to physical activity. After two years, the nondieters had increased their physical activity, reduced their blood pressure and cholesterol, and improved their self-esteem. Their weight remained the same.

By comparison, the dieters initially lost weight and had lower blood pressure, but the improvements didn't last. And their self-esteem declined.

Perhaps most striking, a full 42 percent of the dieters dropped out of the study, while only 8 percent of the nondieters did so. In short, the research suggests that when people stop striving for a body that's unattainable, they're likely to put greater—and more sustained—effort into taking care of the one they have.

WEIGHING BENEFITS AND RISKS

If you decide to go on a diet, remember that despite all the promises from diet-plan pushers, no special menu of foods has been proven to produce long-term weight loss. In fact, a *Consumer Reports* survey of people who successfully lost weight and kept it off found that 83 percent did so on their own without following any particular plan. Whatever method you choose, make sure it doesn't restrict healthful foods and does put an emphasis on physical activity. Above all, keep in mind that dieting isn't guaranteed to make you healthier and may involve risks. Successful weight loss is likely going to require some kind of sacrifice. Just make sure it doesn't include your health—or your life.

TRUSTWORTHY SOURCES OF INFORMATION

The Volumetrics Eating Plan: Techniques and Recipes for Feeling Full on Fewer Calories, by Barbara Rolls (New York: Morrow, 2005). Rolls, a leading authority on weight management, offers an excellent alternative to typical diet books. Her sensible, science-based guide tells how to choose healthful foods that are filling and have fewer calories.

Active Living Every Day, by Steven Blair, Andrea Dunn, Bess Marcus, Ruth Ann Carpenter, and Peter Jaret (Champaign, Ill.: Human Kinetics, 2001). This evidence-based book presents a twenty-week plan to help readers become more physically active. Rather than requiring vigorous exercise, it allows you to choose forms of activity you enjoy and helps you overcome barriers to getting started and sticking with your fitness routine.

Mindless Eating: Why We Eat More Than We Think, by Brian Wansink (New York: Bantam, 2006). Wansink, a prominent food researcher, draws on his own experiments and those of others to provide entertaining insights into our eating habits and offers tips on how to healthfully lose weight without feeling deprived.

Cartoon courtesy www.danscartoons.com

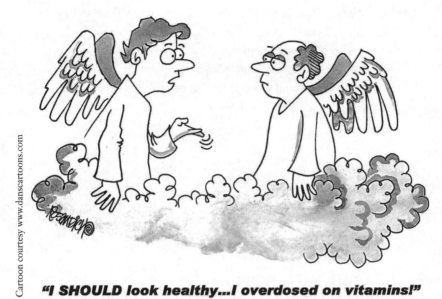

"I SHOULD look healthy...I overdosed on vitamins!"

CHAPTER FOUR: ADVERTISEMENTS
TAKE A SUPPLEMENT!

You are greatly uninformed and should do more research!" screams the e-mail in my inbox. "Don't be so fast to pooh-pooh something you don't embrace or really understand." Scolds another: "Caveats to the impressionable readers who will obviously be duped by your lack of knowledge." So goes the mail, it seems, whenever I report on dietary supplements and raise questions about their claims. I've come to expect it.

On days I receive these howlers—and on just about every other—it's equally predictable that my inbox will also contain ads for supplements of one kind or another. I'm guaranteed to feel better, live longer, get stronger, boost my memory, or ward off disease simply by popping a pill. I'm also told it's possible to magically burn fat and melt away pounds "without changing your eating habits or lifestyle." And then there are the relentless promotions for those penis enlargement and breast enhancement products, promising to "literally change your life."

If you have an e-mail account, odds are that you regularly get spammed with similar promotions for vitamins, minerals, amino acids, and herbs that allegedly promote health and wellness. The vast majority of these claims are baseless, if not blatantly bogus, and deserve to be ignored, which is exactly how most of us respond.

But ads for supplements show up in many other places as well, and because they can't be trapped in a spam filter or instantly obliterated by

pressing the delete key, they're often harder to disregard. Women's magazines, health and fitness publications, and mainstream newspapers frequently carry such advertising, lending it an air of credibility, as do TV
shows and radio programs featuring popular personalities. And sometimes
we're unwittingly the targets of supplement advertising that's cleverly
embedded in what seems to be objective health information.

Whether we admit it or not, such advertising can and does have an
impact. Spending on supplements totals more than $23 billion a year, and
no industry that large survives and thrives on word of mouth alone. Yet the
protections we have against misleading advertising for prescription and
over-the-counter drugs don't apply to the promotion of dietary supplements. The federal government only loosely regulates supplement manufacturers' claims, contrary to popular perception. In one survey, more than
half of respondents (including those who were college educated) wrongly
believed that makers of supplements "are not allowed to make claims for
their safety or effectiveness unless there is solid scientific evidence to support them."

While some ads provide useful and truthful information, many others—
including those for seemingly noncontroversial products such as certain
vitamins—stretch the truth, misleadingly wrapping themselves in the man-
tle of solid science. The rampant deception in supplement marketing
doesn't mean all products are worthless and should be shunned. Indeed,
some can be beneficial. But distinguishing truth from fiction in these marketing claims requires a skeptical eye trained to know what to look for.
Though some supplement enthusiasts such as my angry pen pals may consider this wariness a sign of being "uninformed" or "duped," it's actually evidence of just the opposite.

LAX LAWS

If there were a poster child for the inadequacy of federal regulation regarding dietary supplements, it would have to be the heavily advertised herb
ephedra. Touted as a weight loss aid and a performance enhancer for athletes, the compound—also known as ma huang—acts like an ampheta-
mine, increasing blood pressure and heart rate and decreasing appetite.

Over the years, the herb has been linked to more than 150 deaths as well as serious adverse events, including heart attacks, strokes, and seizures, many in young people. But it wasn't until the highly publicized death of 23-year-old Baltimore Orioles pitcher Steve Bechler, an ephedra user, that the Food and Drug Administration was finally emboldened to yank the herb off the market. As a result, the ubiquitous Internet ads for ephedra products largely disappeared, too.

It took years for the FDA to act because its authority is severely constrained under a law known as the Dietary Supplement Health and Education Act (DSHEA). Passed by Congress in 1994 under intense pressure from the supplement industry, which warned that overzealous government regulators would usurp Americans' freedom to buy vitamins, the law does not require supplement makers to demonstrate that their products are safe or effective before selling them. As long as manufacturers don't explicitly say their products can treat, cure, or prevent illness, they're free to claim pretty much anything they want. (The same rule governs claims for foods, as discussed in chapter 2.) The burden is on the government to prove that a supplement is unsafe. In essence, the law assumes that supplements are innocent until proven guilty—exactly the opposite of how prescription and over-the-counter drugs are regulated. Or, as nutrition expert Marion Nestle puts it, the law rests on "two quite questionable assumptions: that supplements are basically harmless and that supplement makers are honest."

After assembling mounds of evidence about the hazards of ephedra—and nearly ten years after sounding the first alarm—the FDA finally had enough ammunition under the law to ban ephedra products in 2004. Or so it thought. Supplement makers immediately challenged the action in court, and, a year later, they won a partial victory. A federal judge in Utah ruled that the FDA, in arguing that ephedra is not known to be safe at any dose, failed to provide sufficient evidence under DSHEA that low-dose ephedra products were harmful. As a result, ephedra—a demonstrably dangerous substance—could once again be sold legally, as long as supplements contained 10 mg or less of it.

Eventually, the FDA's total ban was upheld, but in the meantime, ephedra ads returned with a vengeance. "EPHEDRA IS BACK!" proclaimed one, describing it as "the herb that was once banned for being TOO effective."

Furthering its fabrication, the Internet ad claimed that since being "taken off the shelves for further testing," the supplement had "gone through rigorous tests" for safety and "passed with flying colors."

Those highly misleading statements were bad enough, but they paled in comparison to the ad's outlandish assertions about ephedra's effectiveness. By taking the product, according to the ad, you will

"slam through your work day"
"be the life of the party"
"be awesome at the gym"
"cure your hangover"
"enhance sexual pleasure"
"lose weight quickly and safely"
"excell [*sic*] in everything you do"

These laughably exaggerated claims were accompanied by glowing testimonials from satisfied customers as well as a guarantee that ephedra is "the best energy and/or weight loss product you have ever taken . . . or you can have 100% of your money back."

Because of the laxness of DSHEA regulations, supplement makers seem to believe that they can run ads like this with impunity. And usually they're right. While claims on labels are the responsibility of the FDA, supplement advertising falls under the jurisdiction of another agency, the Federal Trade Commission. The FTC typically defers to the FDA regarding claims about safety and effectiveness, but in some cases its standards for what is permissible are even more lenient than those of the DSHEA-constrained FDA.

What's more, the FTC is woefully outmatched by supplement hucksters. Faced with an avalanche of misleading supplement ads, especially on the Internet, the commission lacks the staff resources to pursue the vast majority of them. From among the thousands and thousands of supplement ads, the agency has managed to crack down on only a handful, which usually represent the most egregious offenses. Among them:

TV infomercials for two weight loss products, Fat Trapper and Exercise in a Bottle, which claim that users can burn calories "even while resting" and will "never, ever, ever, ever have to diet again."

Magazine and tabloid newspaper ads for PediaLean, a weight loss product for children boasting "a success rate of 100%!"

Direct mail ads for GH3 Romanian Youth Formula, which supposedly lets users live "an average of 29% longer than the normal life expectancy."

Radio ads for a memory-boosting potion called Focus Factor that allegedly lets you "absorb information in books like a sponge."

While trumpeting their toughness against offenders like these, FTC officials admit that there's only so much they can do. "We obviously must make some difficult choices in selecting cases to prosecute," said former commissioner Sheila Anthony in a speech, adding with almost comic understatement, "I worry that . . . there are many unsubstantiated product claims that are going unchallenged." The commission has called on media organizations to be more responsible and refuse supplement ads that make unproven claims. But its appeals have gone largely unheeded.

"CLINICALLY PROVEN"

Though no law requires that supplements be tested for effectiveness, some manufacturers fund research and use it to make marketing claims that their products have been "scientifically studied" or "clinically proven" to work. But typically such research is far too preliminary to provide any real proof of effectiveness. Like some of the studies supported by the food industry, these may be conducted only in test tubes or on animals. Or they may be short-term human experiments involving a small numbers of subjects with no control group. Some of this research involves scientific methods that are highly dubious, if not unethical. For example, lawsuits filed against ephedra supplement makers revealed that companies persuaded researchers to pick and choose data in a way that yielded favorable results for the tested products.

In many cases, "clinically proven" claims are based on research done on other products, which may contain different ingredients. Sometimes those other products aren't even supplements. Consider, for instance, ads for human growth hormone (GH) supplements, promoted to combat aging and reduce weight. Many boast of the following results from a study:

Body fat loss	82 percent improvement
Wrinkle reduction	61 percent improvement
Energy level	84 percent improvement
Muscle strength	88 percent improvement
Sexual potency	75 percent improvement
Emotional stability	67 percent improvement
Memory	62 percent improvement

It turns out that this research involved not the supplements being advertised—and not even other supplements—but prescription growth hormone, which is administered by injection and is far more potent than any supplement. (More on GH in chapter 9.) But it can be tough to figure this out because the ads often fail to list a source for the data they present. And when one is provided, it's sometimes inaccurate (mangling the name of one of the researchers) and incomplete (neglecting to say where the study was published). Further, nearly all the ads give the erroneous impression that the listed percentages reflect the degree of improvement in each area. In fact, they indicate the percentage of patients who reported improvements on questionnaires. The study included no objective measurements to validate the self-reports, and about 80 percent of the subjects either didn't respond or had their answers excluded. Nor was there a control group. In short, these findings provide no "clinical proof" about the effects of GH injections, much less of supplements.

A far more rigorous GH study, this one published in the *New England Journal of Medicine*, is also frequently referenced in supplement ads, with statements such as "Experts in the *New England Journal of Medicine* report that Human Growth Hormone therapy makes you look and feel 20 YEARS YOUNGER!" Like the other study, this one involved injections, not supplements; and the ad's characterization of the researchers' conclusions—which were quite cautious and emphasized the need for far more research—takes them out of context. The journal's editor, denouncing the use of this research to promote GH supplements, wrote in 2003 that if consumers buy products based on this study, "they are being misled." Yet the ads continue, and so do sales.

In addition to citing studies—and sometimes in lieu of it—ads may try to make a scientific case for the product by presenting testimonials from doctors or scientists. Most of these "experts" are paid by manufacturers, and some have highly questionable credentials. Testimonials from product users—another frequent feature of supplement ads—don't add up to evidence, no matter how many are provided or how persuasive they may seem.

Then there's the tactic of arguing that a substance is "time tested"—that its use for hundreds or thousands of years, typically in some faraway place, serves as evidence that it works. For example, a Web site promoting the African herb hoodia has this to say under the heading "The Science behind Hoodia Gordonii": "Is there evidence that Hoodia Gordonii works as an appetite suppressant? Yes! For thousands of years the Bushmen of South Africa having [sic] been eating Hoodia Gordonii to fight off hunger during their long hunting trips. . . . So while the Bushmen did not do formal clinical studies, there is [sic] thousands of years of real world evidence that eating Hoodia suppresses your appetite."

What the ad calls "real world evidence" is, in fact, merely supposition. Because no formal research has been conducted among the Bushmen, it's impossible to know whether this effect (if it exists) is a result of their hoodia use or some other factor. And the fact that the herb has been popular for thousands of years proves nothing about its worth. After all, the medical therapy of bleeding sick people (sometimes to death) was popular for thousands of years, too; and the "science" of astrology, which has been around since antiquity, is still alive and well. Yet neither has scientific merit. Any claim that a supplement works because it is "time tested" ought to be viewed in this light and ignored.

"ALL NATURAL"

The term "natural," a favorite of supplement marketers, is typically used to imply that the product is safe. For example, ads for herbal colon cleansers, which supposedly flush out toxic fecal matter decaying inside the body, frequently describe these products as "all natural" and "safe." What ads for such cleansers don't tell you is that some of their commonly found herbal ingredients, such as cascara sagrada, senna, and rhubarb, are powerful laxatives that can cause cramping and other digestive discomfort. Over time, the colon can become dependent on them for bowel movements. Even more seriously, when taken regularly, these ingredients can lead to harmful or even life-threatening mineral imbalances. Users often unknowingly assume such risks in pursuit of unproven benefits based on the long-debunked theory (espoused by John Harvey Kellogg) that poisons build up inside the body and need to be flushed out by laxatives. A far more natural—and safe—way to stay regular and healthy is a high-fiber diet rich in whole grains, fruits, and vegetables, along with plenty of fluids and regular exercise.

If a substance is powerful enough to have the kinds of therapeutic effects claimed by manufacturers, it is also strong enough to cause unwanted effects in some people. If it never causes any side effects in any users—a claim made for many products—odds are that it's too weak to have a benefit. Yet supplement promoters sometimes try to have it both ways, touting their products as both highly effective and risk-free. What they're implicitly saying is that their products, by virtue of being "natural," aren't governed by basic laws of biology, which, of course, is nonsense.

Supplement proponents are quick to point to the highly publicized side effects of certain prescription medications and to contrast those with the relatively small number of reported risks for "natural" products. But it's a faulty and deceptive comparison. We hear so much about the side effects of prescription drugs because the law requires research and disclosure of risks. Though the system certainly isn't perfect, it does result in an abundance of information about risks and side effects—sometimes more than we want— distributed through product labels, advertisements, and FDA warnings. The lack of such information for supplements doesn't necessarily mean that the products are safer; it just means that we're in the dark about them.

Ads for "natural" products frequently include the line "no known side effects." This artful wording, which implies that no problems exist, actually means none have been detected so far. And when you're not looking very hard (or aren't looking at all), you're unlikely to find anything.

Sometimes the only way to uncover harmful effects, especially long-term ones, is through large clinical trials. That's the lesson of beta-carotene. For years, there was widespread enthusiasm for the supplement, after numerous epidemiological studies suggested that people with higher intakes (mainly through food) had lower rates of cancer and heart disease. The main known side effect was a harmless yellowing of the skin. But two randomized trials involving tens of thousands of people revealed something more: that smokers who took beta-carotene supplements were more likely to develop lung cancer and had higher death rates (heart-related and overall) than those who took a placebo. Without these two studies, many smokers undoubtedly would have continued to pop this supposedly "safe" supplement, unwittingly putting themselves at even greater risk of disease.

In the face of limited science, we often give supplements the benefit of any doubts and assume that their "natural" status makes them safe. That's a mistake. If supplement ads tempt you to fall for this fallacy, remember that many pharmaceuticals with potent side effects come from plants. And don't forget about poisonous mushrooms and hemlock: they're natural, too.

"CAL, AS IN CALCIUM . . ."

Even types of supplements that are generally recognized as legitimate and safe, such as certain vitamins and minerals, are sometimes marketed in misleading ways. Consider, for example, calcium supplements. One popular brand, Citracal, has been heavily promoted on the radio by personalities such as Rush Limbaugh, Dr. Laura Schlessinger, and, most notably, the legendary Paul Harvey, who reaches an estimated 15 million listeners a week. Any regular Harvey listener can likely recite his slogan for the product: "Cit as in citrus, cal as in calcium. Cit-ra-cal." The mellifluous master of the dramatic pause, long a pitchman for a number of products, is credited by the makers of Citracal for boosting sales. "He has a way of taking the essence of any product," the company's president has been quoted as saying, "and putting it across in a conversational manner that rings true with consumers."

But some of what "rings true" in Harvey's ads is in fact hyperbole. Claiming that "every day we learn some new health benefit from Citracal," he tells listeners that not only can it "help fight off the ravages of osteoporosis," but it also promotes heart health and helps control weight. The supplement is "good for you generally," he says, making it sound like some kind of all-around elixir.

Harvey urges us to "keep taking care of ourselves by eating right, exercising regularly, and not smoking, and taking Citracal every day." To borrow a line from the old *Sesame Street* song, one of these things is not like the others. While the benefits of a healthful diet, regular exercise, and not smoking are indisputable, the evidence regarding calcium supplements isn't always so clear-cut. And Harvey's suggestion that the Citracal brand alone confers these purported benefits—he implores listeners, "Please don't gamble with some store brand"—makes his messages all the more misleading.

When it comes to calcium and heart health, a study from New Zealand showed that postmenopausal women who took Citracal for a year had a greater increase in their HDL cholesterol levels than those getting a placebo. But other research has found calcium to have no effect on cholesterol. Given the mixed findings and limited research to date, it's certainly premature to conclude, as Harvey does, that Citracal is "clinically tested and proved good for your heart." His statements regarding weight loss are on similarly shaky ground. As evidence, he points to studies from the University of Tennessee—the same ones the dairy industry has funded and cited to support its questionable claim that milk and other dairy products promote weight loss (as described in chapter 2).

The effects of calcium on bone health have been studied far more extensively, but, once again, the results aren't as definitive as Harvey's ads would have us believe. In a study of nearly 1,500 healthy postmenopausal women, subjects who took Citracal had greater increases in bone density than those who got a placebo. But overall, those who took calcium didn't have fewer bone fractures, which is what really matters. And, surprisingly, they were *more* likely to break their hips. The authors concluded that the effect of calcium on fractures "remains uncertain."

Various efforts to pool data from multiple studies—a technique known as meta-analysis—have resulted in conflicting conclusions about whether calcium (either alone or with vitamin D, which helps the body absorb calcium) reduces the risk of fractures. And the Women's Health Initiative, a trial of 36,000 women that was expected to provide definitive answers, failed to do so. Overall, those who took calcium and vitamin D for seven years did not have fewer broken bones than those who took a placebo, although some subsets of women (those who were older and those who took their pills more regularly) did have slightly fewer fractures. Summing up the evidence, one expert wrote that "any benefit of calcium plus vitamin D on bone mineral density or the risk of fracture is, at best, small and may vary from group to group."

So while calcium supplements may be beneficial for certain people, the pills don't deserve to be billed as a proven health measure for the entire population, akin to exercise and not smoking. And, despite what Paul Harvey implies, there's nothing unique about Citracal that makes it better for your overall health than comparable brands of calcium.

MULTI-CLAIM MULTIVITAMINS

You can also find plenty of questionable advertising claims for multivitamins, the most popular category of supplements. At one time, all multivitamins were pretty much the same, providing 100 percent of the recommended amounts of most vitamins and minerals. But no more. Today, with countless multis competing for market share, manufacturers are increasingly touting their products as specially designed for particular populations or health needs. You can find multis targeted at not only men, women, and seniors but also smokers, dieters, diabetics, and even teachers.

One company, GenSpec Labs, makes and markets what it calls "genetically specific" multis that are supposedly tailored for various ethnic and racial groups. Among the eye-grabbing ads for the supplements is one that appears in African American publications, showing a buff black man in a pink tutu surrounded by white girls in ballet outfits. In large letters, it asks, "Have you been taking someone else's vitamins?" In smaller print, the ad explains that "African American men have a greater nutritional need to regulate blood sugar, address prostate health, maintain a healthy heart, kidney and weight control" and that GenSpec is formulated "to address these genetically specific health concerns."

This formulation includes a slew of extra ingredients such as rutin powder, green tea extract, and lycopene. But the evidence for their effectiveness tends to be preliminary at best, and the limited research that exists typically involves higher levels than those found in the GenSpec multis.

Further, doses of many vitamins and minerals in the GenSpec supplements for black men exceed the government's recommended daily values (DVs). Amounts of vitamin E, for example, add up to ten times the DV. Research involving Finnish smokers found that those who took supple-

ments containing 2.5 times the DV for vitamin E had lower rates of prostate cancer than men who took placebos. Prostate cancer is of special concern to African American men because they are more likely than others to
develop and die from it. But it remains unproven that the level of vitamin
E in GenSpec—or any level—is ideal for protecting black men.

Likewise, it's not clear that the supplements' large doses of other nutrients
provide any additional benefits beyond the DVs—whether for African
Americans or anyone else. There's no evidence they cause harm, either.
However, those who take mega-dose multis and also consume fortified foods
and beverages may end up exceeding the safe upper limits for certain nutrients. The result can be problems ranging from diarrhea to kidney stones to
hip fractures. (To get information on safe upper limits for various vitamins
and minerals, along with possible adverse effects, see the Trustworthy
Sources section at the end of the chapter.)

The misguided notion that if some is good, more must be better also
seems to underlie the marketing of multivitamins intended to decrease
stress or boost energy. Take, for example, TV ads for One-A-Day All-Day
Energy Vitamins, which claim that the product's higher levels of B vitamins
(200 percent of the DV) "help you feel energized all day." Similarly, com-
mercials for Centrum Performance multivitamins tell us that "unlike ordinary multivitamins, Centrum Performance is charged with higher levels of
energy-essential nutrients to help re-energize your body every day."

Such ads misleadingly imply that vitamins are a source of energy. In
fact, we get energy from the calories in food, not from vitamins. It's true
that certain B vitamins are essential for turning carbohydrates from food
into energy, and deficiencies of these vitamins can interfere with normal
functioning and cause harm. But for some of these B vitamins (including
thiamine and riboflavin), it's relatively easy to get sufficient amounts from
our diet; for others, a supplement containing 100 percent of the DV is adequate to do the job. There's no proof that extra amounts will make you feel
more energetic. Nor is there hard evidence for Centrum's claim that when
you're under stress—and who isn't?—your body requires higher than recommended levels of vitamins.

If the All-Day Energy multis give you a boost, it's probably because they
also contain caffeine. But you wouldn't know this from the ads, which

instead refer to something called an "extended-release guarana blend." In fact, guarana is a tropical plant with high levels of caffeine, and the "blend" consists of guarana powder plus more caffeine. A more apt name would be "caffeine buzz blend."

Whether multis are specially targeted or not, ads for them often imply— and sometimes say explicitly—that the products will help keep you healthy. In reality, the jury is still out on the benefits of multivitamins. A panel of experts convened by the National Institutes of Health concluded that the evidence was insufficient to recommend either for or against their use to prevent disease. But it certainly may make sense to take a basic multi as a form of insurance, especially if you are older, a heavy drinker, a smoker, a vegetarian, or a dieter severely restricting calories. Also, a multi can help ensure that women who are pregnant or might become pregnant get adequate amounts of folic acid, which has been shown to prevent neural-tube birth defects. Still, no multivitamin can make up for a bad diet, no matter how high its levels of vitamins and minerals or how many extra ingredients are thrown in.

STEALTH MARKETING

Sometimes the marketing of supplements comes in disguised forms. One example is certain genetic tests marketed directly to consumers as a tool for providing individualized nutrition and lifestyle guidance. Typically, consumers receive a kit with a cheek swab and instructions for obtaining a DNA sample; they then send the sample to the company's lab. Test results, which supposedly identify genetic deficiencies that increase susceptibility to disease, are in some cases accompanied by recommendations for specific dietary supplements—products the test manufacturers just happen to sell. One such company says it offers "a personalized protocol of specially formulated nutraceuticals that interact with your body's own DNA repair processes, and provide targeted, high-density genetic nourishment."

While scientific-sounding language like this may seem compelling, it's in fact a lot of hot air. That's basically the conclusion of an investigation by the Government Accountability Office (GAO), which purchased genetic tests from four Web sites and submitted DNA samples for fourteen fictitious consumers of various ages, weights, and lifestyles. The GAO found that the supposedly "personalized" supplement recommendations were the same for everyone, whether the individual was a 72-year-old female nonsmoker with a high-protein diet or a 45-year-old male smoker with a high-fat diet. One site recommended a nutritional formula containing vitamins and minerals typically found in a multivitamin—but at the exorbitant price of about $1,200 for a one-year supply. By contrast, a comparable product you'd find at the grocery store costs $35 a year, according to the GAO.

Another company's recommended regimen, which ran nearly $1,900 a year, included the herb cat's claw and other ingredients that allegedly help repair DNA. In fact, there's no evidence that any supplement can do this. There is concern, however, that cat's claw may interact with blood-thinning medications and increase the risk of bleeding. Nutrition experts consulted by the GAO investigators also pointed out that some of the recommended supplements contained excessive and potentially harmful levels of vitamin A and iron.

These testing companies overstate the connections among genes, nutrition, and health, making them appear far stronger and better understood than they actually are. When offered by supplement sellers, testing serves as bait to seduce us into buying. Far from getting supplements tailored to our particular genetic makeup, as if such a thing were even possible, we may end up with overpriced products that we don't need.

Sneaky sales pitches are also what you get at the Web site of Dr. Andrew Weil, one of the nation's most prominent and trusted experts on dietary supplements. With his best-selling books and ubiquitous media presence, the guru of "integrative medicine" (which combines conventional and alternative methods) has attracted a large and loyal following of people who look to him for sensible, evenhanded advice about which vitamins, minerals, and herbs are—and are not—worth trying.

Weil's Web site, drweil.com, promises to personalize the good doctor's guidance. "Confused about vitamins?" it asks. "Let Dr. Weil help." Clicking the link takes you to a service called Vitamin Advisor, which invites you to answer questions about your health history and lifestyle and receive free individualized recommendations regarding which supplements you need.

Sounds great. But this seemingly objective source of information is actually a tool for peddling Weil's own line of supplements, described as "exclusive formulas developed for maximum effectiveness." When I completed the online questionnaire, the site suggested that I—a healthy male in my 40s who exercises regularly and eats a healthful diet—take Dr. Weil's anti-oxidant and multivitamin formula, which consists of levels of some vitamins and minerals that are more than 1,000 percent of the recommended daily values. On top of that, I was told to take several other supplements, includ-ing one containing omega-3 (fish oil), a B-vitamin complex for "vessel sup-port," and something called "environmental support," which is 2,000 mg of vitamin C for people who live in cities with air pollution. (Never mind that Weil himself says the body cannot use more than about 250 mg of vita-min C a day.) The price tag for all these pills (eight a day, to be exact): more than $65 a month, or nearly $800 a year. Someone with more health issues would undoubtedly have an even lengthier, more expensive list of recom-mendations.

According to an investigation by the Center for Science in the Public Interest, Weil has raked in several million dollars as part of a five-year, $14 million deal he signed in 2003 with drugstore.com to sell his supple-ments. (The agreement was later renegotiated after drugstore.com sued Weil.) Weil says all after-tax proceeds go into his nonprofit foundation, which supports research and education in integrative medicine. How the money is used or how much he makes is beside the point, though. What matters is that this trusted doctor has a vested interest in consumers buying his supple-ments. The more he sells, the more he earns for his causes, an arrangement that calls into question the objectivity of his personalized recommendations. Though the site claims that "the Vitamin Advisor is not about products," the fact that it pushes Weil's supplements suggests otherwise. When consulting the site, consumers would do well to heed the wise advice that Weil offers elsewhere about supplements: *"caveat emptor*—buyer beware!"

EQUAL-OPPORTUNITY SKEPTICISM

So how do we translate that old axiom into action when confronted with claims in supplement ads? Keeping a few key guidelines in mind can help:

- VERIFY "CLINICALLY PROVEN" CLAIMS. If a reference to a published study is provided, look it up on PubMed.gov. At the very least, make sure it's relevant to the product and was a randomized human trial. If there's no reference or if the research is unpublished, contact the company and ask to get a copy of the study. If the manufacturer can't or won't comply, consider it a red flag.

- DON'T ASSUME THAT "NATURAL" MEANS SAFE. Instead, check out supplements as you would any other drug and look for a list of possible side effects and contraindications on the package or the product's Web site. If no list exists, consider the possibility that the supplement hasn't been sufficiently tested or that the manufacturer has something to hide.

- BE SKEPTICAL OF CLAIMS THAT A SOUPED-UP OR SPECIALLY TARGETED VITAMIN OR MINERAL SUPPLEMENT IS BETTER THAN AN ORDINARY ONE. Read labels carefully to see what's different, and watch out for multis with mega-doses of vitamins and minerals or with added herbs and other ingredients.

- DON'T BE SWAYED BY WEASEL WORDS. Phrases such as "maintains heart health" or "provides immune support" may imply that the product can prevent heart disease or ward off infections, but such words are actually meaningless. Supplement makers use this kind of fuzzy phrasing (as opposed to explicitly saying that something prevents or treats a condition) because under law they don't have to back it up with evidence.

- BE WARY OF ORGANIZATIONS OR INDIVIDUALS WHO PROVIDE INFORMATION ABOUT SUPPLEMENTS AND ALSO SELL THEM. Instead, look for recommendations from objective sources with no financial ties to the supplement industry.

Above all, let science and reason be your guide, not ideology, emotion, or faith. Some who use supplements embrace them out of a deep distrust of the pharmaceutical industry, believing that drug companies deceitfully market harmful products and even conspire with the government and the media to suppress and discredit dietary supplements. While such views are clearly open to debate, let's assume for argument's sake that they're true. Should we then automatically trust supplement makers, who, after all, are also trying to sell us something (and in some cases are part of pharmaceutical companies)? Why should they be subject to any less skepticism and scrutiny? Instead of thinking of "bad guys" (drug companies) versus "good guys" (supplement makers), we need to be equal-opportunity skeptics and demand solid scientific evidence from everyone regarding safety and effectiveness. Those who can't or won't convincingly back up their advertising claims, regardless of whether their pills are "natural" or not, don't deserve our trust—or our business.

TRUSTWORTHY SOURCES OF INFORMATION

Natural Medicines Comprehensive Database (www.consumerreports .org/health/natural-medicine/index.htm). This resource provides evidence-based information regarding the effectiveness, safety, and possible interactions of more than 14,000 vitamins, herbs, and other dietary supplements. The database, offered by *Consumer Reports,* was created by the Therapeutic Research Center, which independently analyzes medications and supplements. There is a small fee to access the information.

The "Drugs and Supplements" section on the Mayo Clinic's Web site (www.mayoclinic.com/health/drug-information/HerbIndex/). This includes excellent background information on a host of dietary supplements, along with an evaluation of the evidence (graded on a scale of A to F) for specific uses. It also provides dosing and safety information. The database comes from Natural Standard, an independent group that impartially evaluates evidence for alternative and complementary therapies.

ConsumerLab.com. This organization tests dietary supplements to determine whether they in fact contain what's listed on the label, are free of impurities, and break down properly in the body. Complete reports, which include test results plus useful background information on various types of products, are available through the group's Web site for a subscription fee.

Dietary Reference Intake tables (www.iom.edu/CNS/3788/7292 .aspx). The tables list age- and gender-specific recommended daily values for vitamins and minerals, as determined by the Institute of Medicine. Included are safe upper limits, effects of excess consumption, and food sources.

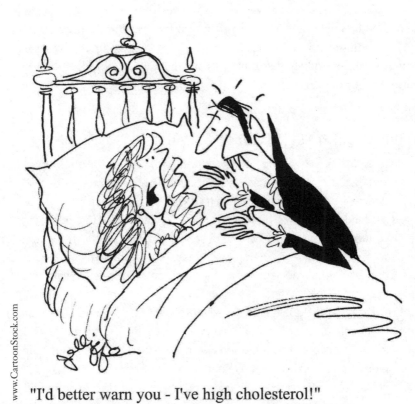

www.CartoonStock.com

"I'd better warn you - I've high cholesterol!"

CHAPTER FIVE: GOVERNMENT CAMPAIGNS
WATCH YOUR CHOLESTEROL!

My friend Mrs. F. worked hard to stay healthy, and it showed. Well into her 80s, she walked several miles a day, watched what she ate, and weighed the same as she had as a young woman. She was largely free of the aches, pains, and infirmities that afflicted many of her contemporaries. Possessing boundless energy and intense curiosity about others, she could have easily passed for someone 15 years her junior. In short, she had every reason to be content about her health. But she wasn't. Whenever I asked how she felt, I invariably got the same response. "You know," she would say in her deep southern drawl, her voice dropping to a confessional whisper, "I have high cholesterol." Her doctor had put her on medication to lower it.

Though I always tried to suggest that she probably shouldn't be too worried about it, I knew my assurances were in vain. Consistent with ubiquitous public health warnings, Mrs. F. believed that she had a condition that could kill her and that she must remain vigilant. The truth, however, is that high cholesterol is not a condition or a disease. As studies have shown, it's one factor among many that may raise the risk of heart disease *for certain people*—but perhaps not for healthy 85-year-old women. What's more, the medication Mrs. F. was taking to treat this "condition" may pose risks that outweigh any possible benefits in people like her.

If you don't know a Mrs. F., perhaps you're acquainted with someone like Mr. G. He's a 50-year-old couch potato whose idea of exercise is lifting the remote to switch channels. More often than not, his meals consist of a burger and fries for lunch and pizza for dinner. He has high blood pressure, smokes a pack of cigarettes a day, and is under enormous stress from his job. If you suggest that he should try to take better care of himself, he acknowledges that his health habits aren't perfect but says recent test results give him reason not to worry: he has low cholesterol.

Because of relentless messages about the hazards of high cholesterol, Mr. G. has gotten the misimpression that cholesterol level trumps everything else in determining susceptibility to a heart attack. What Mr. G. doesn't realize is that half of those who suffer heart attacks have normal cholesterol levels. Despite his cholesterol reading, he's a prime candidate for a heart attack because of his other risk factors. He has every reason to be concerned.

The misguided views of Mrs. F., Mr. G., and millions of others like them are largely the unintended consequence of a massive campaign by the federal government to raise awareness about the importance of cholesterol. Unquestionably, it's been a big success in achieving its goals: more people are aware of cholesterol, and more doctors are prescribing cholesterol-lowering treatments.

The problem is that the campaign's intensive focus on high cholesterol has bestowed it with an undeservedly exalted status—a *primus alter pares* among risk factors for heart disease or, as *Time* magazine put it, a "well-earned reputation as the heart's primary nemesis." Implying that our risk of heart disease can be boiled down to a simple score, this view leads many to put too much stock in their cholesterol numbers. Further, the campaign gives the impression that we're all equally at risk from elevated cholesterol—a notion at odds with the scientific evidence—and recommends cholesterol-lowering medication for people who haven't been shown to benefit from it.

This is not to say we should just forget about cholesterol. To the contrary, we should be aware of it. But we need to keep its role—and that of medication—in perspective. Heart health, which is far more complex than cholesterol campaign slogans frequently convey, involves more than knowing a number and popping a pill.

MARKETING MESSAGES

Despite cholesterol's reputation as a villain, it's something our bodies need to function properly. Made in the liver, cholesterol is a key constituent of membranes surrounding cells and is essential to the formation of hormones. Our brains contain relatively large amounts of it. Cholesterol is transported in the blood by compounds called lipoproteins. When there's too much of one particular type, known as low-density lipoprotein, or LDL, it can build up in artery walls and lead to the formation of plaque. Over time, this can narrow the artery and restrict the supply of blood to the heart. If a clot forms, it can block the artery completely, resulting in a heart attack or stroke. High-density lipoprotein, or HDL, is believed to have the opposite effect, taking cholesterol away from the arteries.

In 1985, the National Heart, Lung, and Blood Institute (NHLBI), part of the National Institutes of Health, launched the National Cholesterol Education Program (NCEP). Its mission: to "contribute to reducing illness and death from coronary heart disease (CHD) in the United States by reducing the percent of Americans with high blood cholesterol." At the time, about 25 percent of American adults had high cholesterol (defined by the NCEP as a total reading of 240 mg/dL or above), and more than half had levels above the "desirable" cutoff of 200 mg/dL. The program therefore needed to get the attention of tens of millions of people, who in many cases would require medical supervision to lower their levels. As NCEP director Dr. James Cleeman put it, "It's a mammoth intervention, and it deserves to be a mammoth intervention."

This intervention targets both the general public and health professionals. Educational efforts aimed at the public have relied on what's known as social marketing, a commonly used strategy that involves applying techniques from commercial marketing to the "selling" of ideas, attitudes, and behaviors. Instead of shoes or televisions, the "products" being sold in this case are the notions that high cholesterol can lead to heart disease, that it's important to know your number, and that you can take steps to lower it. To help plan and execute this sales effort, the NCEP has hired leading public relations firms, which have crafted campaign messages and slogans.

A key part of the sales strategy has been public service advertisements stressing the importance of knowing your cholesterol number. "The higher the number, the higher your risk of heart disease," said a typical print message. "Find out your cholesterol number. And ask your doctor what it means to you." Another ad, using fear to spur us to action, told us, "Heart disease will kill 500,000 people this year. They won't be selected at random." At the bottom was the tag line: "Do you know your cholesterol level?"

A television ad from the early days of the campaign showed a hand operating a water pump, as the unnerving sound of a thumping heart continued relentlessly in the background. "There is a major cause of heart attacks that can affect anyone, no matter who they are: high blood cholesterol," said the announcer, whose ominous tone sounded like something out of a preview for a suspense film. Telling us there may be no symptoms, he warned, "Most likely it's doing its share of damage," at which point a clogged pipe appeared. We then learned what we could do to head off this threat: "Have your cholesterol level checked, and find out what your number means to you."

Other, less foreboding TV spots offered a similar take-home message. One, for example, was a cartoon of Benjamin Franklin flying kites with cholesterol readings on them. "Anyone can have a cholesterol number that's high," said the announcer. "In other words, if your cholesterol number is too high, you could have a heart attack or worse." Like other ads, this one ended with the text line "Know your cholesterol number."

Without question, messages like these have sunk in. By 1990, nearly all American adults—93 percent of those surveyed—had heard of high cholesterol, up from 77 percent before the NCEP's educational efforts began. In a 2001 survey, more than 85 percent of respondents said it was very or extremely important to have healthy cholesterol levels. The proportion of people getting tested in the previous 5 years—another measure of the campaign's success—has increased substantially since 1986, from less than half to about 70 percent in 2006. Meanwhile, average total cholesterol levels have declined to less than 200, and the percentage of people whose numbers fall in the high range has dropped substantially.

SCIENCE VERSUS SLOGANS

As impressive as these achievements may seem, it's important to remember that cholesterol lowering, in and of itself, is not (or should not be) the ultimate goal. What counts is whether lower cholesterol numbers are reducing the rates of heart disease and early death. Population statistics don't provide a clear answer. While it's true that death rates from heart disease have fallen along with cholesterol levels during the past several decades, it's impossible to tease out cholesterol's precise contribution. Other factors, such as lower smoking rates and better treatments for heart disease, have likely played a role as well.

The NCEP insists that its messages about the dangers of elevated cholesterol and the benefits of lowering it are based "firmly on sound scientific evidence." But a close look at the science reveals that high cholesterol isn't the equal-opportunity threat that the ads portray it to be, nor are low levels always more beneficial.

One study frequently cited by the NCEP is the federally funded Framingham Heart Study, which began in 1948 and continues to this day. As described in chapter 1, researchers gathered health data on 5,000 volunteers from Framingham, Massachusetts—and later their children and grandchildren—following them to document how they fared. The landmark cohort study identified a number of factors associated with a higher risk of heart disease, including elevated cholesterol. Subjects with the highest levels were more likely to experience chest pain, heart attacks, or sudden death.

What's often overlooked—or conveniently ignored—is that the Framingham findings applied only to middle-aged people. As subjects got older, the risk posed by high cholesterol appeared to decline. By age 70, there was no relationship between elevated cholesterol and death from heart disease. At age 80, lower cholesterol was associated with a *higher* risk of death from all causes.

A number of other studies involving different populations have also cast doubt on the dangers of high cholesterol in the elderly. For example, the Cardiovascular Health Study, a multicenter cohort study of nearly 6,000 noninstitutionalized people age 65 and older, found that total and LDL cholesterol levels were not major predictors of strokes, heart attacks, or death. Another cohort study, this one involving residents of New Haven, Connecticut, turned up no connection between cholesterol levels and chest pain, hospitalization from heart attacks, or death among subjects older than 70. Research involving Japanese American men in Hawaii, ages 71 to 93, found *higher* death rates among those with low cholesterol, as did a study of racially mixed older people living in New York City.

The NCEP's public education efforts fail to give older people even an inkling of this evidence. Instead, they target young and old alike with the same one-size-fits-all advice, disseminated through ads and educational materials with slogans such as "cholesterol counts for everyone." The NCEP Web site, proclaiming that "cholesterol lowering is important for young, middle-aged, and older adults," offers the sweeping generalization that "whether you have heart disease or want to prevent it, you can reduce your risk for having a heart attack by lowering your cholesterol level." It also says people over 65 can "benefit greatly from lowering elevated cholesterol" and urges them to "keep their cholesterol low."

Such rhetoric may be causing unnecessary anxiety in some older people. In a survey of healthy people age 65 and older, about half of whom had normal or only mildly elevated cholesterol readings, 59 percent reported being at least slightly worried about their cholesterol. One-third were at least moderately worried. Two-thirds were actively trying to keep their levels down, most often by following a special diet or exercising.

A CHOLESTEROL-CENTRIC WORLDVIEW

Certainly, eating a healthful diet and getting physical activity are highly worthwhile goals. The NCEP, to its credit, promotes both as part of its recommendations for what it calls "therapeutic lifestyle changes" (TLC). But, by and large, it frames such steps narrowly as solutions to high cholesterol, rather than as good health habits everyone should adopt regardless of their cholesterol levels.

An NCEP booklet, for example, explains, "What you eat greatly affects your blood cholesterol levels. That's why a key step in your treatment is to adopt a heart healthy eating plan—one that's low in saturated fat, trans fat, and cholesterol." A more accurate way to put it is that what you eat can greatly affect your *overall health*—including, perhaps, your cholesterol level. Lower cholesterol is not the only possible benefit—or even necessarily the main one—of eating a diet rich in fruits, vegetables, and fiber and low in refined carbohydrates, animal fat, and trans fats. The same goes for exercise. While the booklet touches on some of these other benefits (such as controlling blood pressure and reducing the risk of diabetes), it mentions them only in passing, making them seem secondary. It's quite possible to get the erroneous impression from the NCEP's materials that if your cholesterol isn't high, you have less reason to worry about diet and exercise.

A properly drawn diagram of the heart disease prevention "solar system" would put lifestyle measures such as diet, exercise, and smoking cessation at the center, with various benefits, including lower cholesterol, circling around the core. Like pre-Copernican astronomers, however, the NCEP gets things backward, placing an orbital (cholesterol) at the center and everything else on the periphery. Though this isn't literally how the educational materials characterize things, it's certainly the idea they convey. For example, the NCEP's Web site, listing the risk factors for heart disease that we can do something about, puts high cholesterol at the top, ahead of smoking, high blood pressure, diabetes, and physical inactivity.

The words the NCEP uses to describe cholesterol also sometimes exaggerate its importance. An NCEP pamphlet states that your cholesterol level "has a lot to do with your chances of getting heart disease." Well, that all depends on who "you" are and what "a lot" means. According to the Framingham Risk Assessment Tool, which predicts an individual's chance of developing heart disease based on certain characteristics, a 40-year-old man who has a high cholesterol reading of 240 mg/dL, but no other risk factors and no history of heart disease, has a 2 percent risk of developing heart disease in the next 10 years. The same man with a cholesterol level of 180, which is in the normal range, has a 1 percent risk. Is that difference "a lot"? Most people would say no.

Likewise, a 50-year-old nonsmoking woman without high blood pressure has a 1 percent risk of heart disease if her cholesterol level is elevated and less than a 1 percent risk if it's normal. Again, not much of a difference. But if our example is a 50-year-old man who smokes and has high blood pressure, the picture becomes very different. If his cholesterol is normal, his risk of heart disease is 13 percent—and it shoots up to 22 percent if his cholesterol is high.

As these illustrations show, cholesterol cannot be viewed in isolation. Its potential impact depends on a number of other factors, including age, gender, blood pressure, and smoking. So, when the NCEP makes the blanket statement on its Web site, for example, that "your LDL level is a good indicator of your risk for heart disease," it's not telling us the whole story.

Nor are we well served when the NCEP informs us that high cholesterol is a "serious condition," as it does in educational materials. In fact, there's a big difference between a condition and a risk factor such as elevated cholesterol. The NCEP's rhetoric leads us to wrongly believe that the two are synonymous and that if we have high cholesterol, we have a problem not unlike diabetes, asthma, or arthritis.

This exaggeration is perhaps the inevitable consequence of the NCEP's singular focus on cholesterol. It's also the result of the NCEP's need to get our attention with simple, easy-to-understand messages. We're much more likely to heed warnings about a "serious condition" than about something described (more accurately) as one of many factors that has a variable effect on the risk of heart disease, depending on who you are. Of course, the latter doesn't exactly lend itself to catchy slogans. Characterizing high cholesterol as a condition may help the NCEP succeed in its marketing mission, but it fails to give us the full truth.

DISEASE-MONGERING

Turning high cholesterol into an illness is an example of what some call "disease-mongering"—stretching the definition of disease so that more people get labeled as "sick" and require medical treatment. The late health journalist Lynn Payer, who wrote about this phenomenon in her book *Disease-Mongers*, listed three consequences of labeling risk factors as diseases:

> Risk factors come to be seen as bad even in situations where they pose very little risk to the people who have them.

> People assume that by treating the risk factors, they are preventing disease, which isn't always the case.

> The line between what is normal and what is "high" is frequently drawn in such a way that the maximum number of people are labeled "at risk" and are therefore candidates for medical intervention.

The NCEP has managed to produce all three consequences through not only its public education efforts but also its outreach to health professionals, which includes clinical guidelines on treating high cholesterol. Since 1988, there have been several iterations of these highly influential recommendations, known as Adult Treatment Panels, or ATPs. Devised by committees of experts chosen by the NCEP, the guidelines specify who should be treated and how, and what the goals of therapy should be.

Over time, ATPs have continued to broaden the definition of who needs cholesterol-lowering medications, the most common of which are statins such as Lipitor and Crestor. Under guidelines released in 2001, the eligible population of drug recipients nearly tripled, increasing from 13 million to

36 million. Three years later, it expanded again, when a 2004 NCEP panel called for even more aggressive use of statins, which were already the top-selling class of drugs in the United States.

Before 2004, guidelines had stipulated that people at high risk for heart disease (those who already had cardiovascular disease or diabetes or multiple risk factors) were candidates for medication if their LDL levels were 130 mg/dL or higher. The updated recommendations lowered that threshold to 100 mg/dL and suggested that aiming for less than 70 is a "reasonable clinical strategy" for those at very high risk. Further, for those at moderately high risk (with two or more risk factors), lowering the goal from 130 to 100 was now likewise a "therapeutic option" (a course of action that should be considered). The 2004 guidelines, which applied to men and women of all ages, meant that many people who previously had not been candidates for statins now suddenly were. And those already on statins might need higher doses and possibly an additional drug to meet the targets.

According to the NCEP panel, its updated recommendations were based on the latest evidence from recent clinical trials of statin drugs. But not everyone shared the panel's interpretation of that evidence. More than thirty physicians and research scientists joined the Center for Science in the Public Interest in calling on the National Institutes of Health (of which the NCEP is a part) to re-review the data.

One of their concerns was the possibility—or at least the appearance—of a conflict of interest. Eight of the nine experts who wrote the 2004 update to the guidelines had been recipients of speaking honoraria, research funding, or consulting fees from statin manufacturers.

Defending its selections, the federal government says panelists are chosen for their "scientific and medical expertise, their stature and track record in the field, and their integrity." Indeed, all are respected experts in the field, and there's no proof that their ties to drug makers have directly influenced their views. Nevertheless, the lack of at least a few conflict-free panelists does suggest a dearth of scientific diversity, which can lead to lopsided conclusions. Dr. Jerome Kassirer, a former editor-in-chief of the *New England Journal of Medicine*, explains that "when companies with identical interests are underwriting virtually all the researchers, decision makers can become susceptible to 'group think.' The military has a name for this sort of trap—'incestuous amplification.'"

Large randomized trials have demonstrated that statins can head off heart attacks and delay death in people who already have heart disease—so-called secondary prevention. (Some experts suspect that the benefits may be due more to the drugs' anti-inflammatory effects than to their impact on cholesterol.) But research shows the value of the drugs isn't as clear-cut when it comes to primary prevention—protecting those without heart disease. According to one study, as many as 75 percent of people on statins fall into this category, and the experts who petitioned the National Institutes of Health question the NCEP's guidelines for such individuals.

One of the dissenting doctors, John Abramson of Harvard Medical School, and his colleague Dr. James Wright of the University of British Columbia conducted their own analysis of the research by pooling primary prevention results from eight randomized statin trials. They found that people who took statins had a lower risk of heart attacks and other cardiovascular events than those getting placebos. But, overall, the absolute difference in risk was slight—1.5 percent—meaning that 67 people would have to be treated for five years to prevent one cardiovascular event, according to the authors. What's more, subjects taking statins did not have lower death rates. Dr. Wright believes that if people understood how modest the benefit is, many would say to their doctors, "You're expecting me to take a pill every day for five years? And it's going to cost me two dollars a day? You're crazy! I'm not going to do it."

The benefits of statins appeared greatest in high-risk men ages 30 to 69. Women without heart disease didn't seem to be helped at all by statins, a finding that's consistent with another review of the research. This result could reflect either the limitations of statin trials, which tend to underrepresent women, or the difficulty of detecting benefits in women, whose risk of heart disease is generally lower than that of men. Or it could also be that healthy women don't in fact benefit from statins.

Whatever the case, the NCEP's recommendation that healthy women take statins is based not on direct evidence but on extrapolations from findings in men and in women with heart disease. In his book *Overdosed America*, Dr. Abramson likened the enthusiasm for statins to the push to put millions of women on hormone replacement therapy despite a lack of iron-clad evidence. "Such a sweeping recommendation," he wrote, "without unimpeachable evidence from the gold standard of at least one large randomized clinical trial, and optimally several such trials, makes a travesty of the claim that American medicine upholds its standards of excellence by adhering strictly to scientific evidence."

In their analysis, Abramson and Wright also found that healthy people 70 and older didn't appear to benefit from statins. But because age is a risk factor for heart disease, many older people are considered at least moderately high risk, making them candidates for relatively aggressive therapy under the NCEP's guidelines. Indeed, the number of older people on statins has grown substantially in recent years, with more than 20 percent of those 60 and over on medication—a far higher proportion than among people 40 to 59.

The NCEP argues that, given their elevated risk, the elderly stand to benefit even more than others from cholesterol lowering and that not prescribing statins to them would cost lives. The problem with this logic is that it presupposes a relationship between cholesterol levels and the risk of heart disease in older people. If, as a number of epidemiological studies suggest, high cholesterol ceases to be a risk factor as people get older, then lowering levels—no matter how high the overall risk of heart disease—may be of little use.

If there were no drawbacks to statins, none of these gaps in the evidence would matter too much. The medication could be prescribed as a general wellness measure for nearly everyone—or even put in the water supply, as some enthusiasts have suggested. But, like all other drugs, statins do have potential downsides. For starters, the cost of prescribing them to tens of millions more people is steep, perhaps exceeding $100 billion. Even researchers who believe that healthy people should take the drugs acknowledge that the cost may not be justified in those at intermediate risk and certainly not in those at low risk.

Though statins are widely regarded as relatively safe, they do have possible risks and side effects that need to be considered. One is liver damage, which can be prevented with regular blood tests. A potentially more serious threat is muscle pain and weakness, which manifests itself in different forms, including in rare cases a potentially deadly condition known as rhabdomyolysis. (One statin, Baycol, was withdrawn from the market in 2001 because of this side effect.) People who are over 80 (especially women), as well as those who are frail, have multiple illnesses, or take multiple medications, are more likely to develop muscle problems associated with statins, and they're more likely to be debilitated by them.

In a review of the research, Dr. Beatrice Golomb of the University of California, San Diego, notes that another possible effect in the elderly is impaired memory and thinking. Though the evidence for this particular side effect is mixed—different trials, using different measures, have reached different conclusions—the potential risk needs to be taken seriously in older people, who are more likely to be adversely affected by even small cognitive changes.

Then there's the issue of cancer. A trial involving people age 70 and older reported that those taking statins had a statistically significant 25 percent increase in cancer rates compared to those getting placebos. Ordinarily, such a result would raise red flags and prompt researchers to urge further investigation. But instead, the authors of this study, which was funded by statin manufacturer Bristol-Myers Squibb, went out of their way to exonerate statins, dismissing their own finding as a fluke. Merging their data with those from other trials, they concluded that there was no connection between statins and cancer, a position parroted by the NCEP.

Several other efforts to pool results from multiple studies have also found no increased risk of cancer among statin users. But another such analysis, which included studies that involved more aggressive cholesterol lowering, produced what the researchers called a "disturbing" finding: statin-takers with the lowest LDL levels were more likely to be diagnosed with cancer. This result echoes epidemiological studies that have linked low cholesterol to a higher risk of death from cancer. None of this proves, however, that low LDL or statin use *causes* cancer; it's possible that low cholesterol is a result of previously undiagnosed cancer or that some other unknown factor explains the apparent relationship. Nevertheless, the evidence is sufficient to warrant further research and should at least give pause to those pushing for aggressive cholesterol lowering in healthy people, especially the elderly, who are more prone to develop cancer.

Scientists are only beginning to understand statins' full range of effects (both good and bad) beyond lowering cholesterol. People often must take the drugs for life, and any long-term effects are still unknown. This isn't to say they are unsafe or shouldn't be used. Statins clearly have a role in preventing heart attacks, perhaps even among certain individuals for whom there's less solid evidence of a benefit. But weighing the risks and benefits among healthy people is different than doing so among those with heart disease. Before a statin or any other drug is prescribed preemptively to someone who is well, we must have maximum certainty that the chances of a benefit far outweigh any possibility of harm. Put another way, subjecting those in good health to treatments that could possibly rob them of it is unacceptable without a very compelling reason for doing so.

This basic principle seems to get lost amid the NCEP's zealous promotion of statins for more and more healthy people. Excessive enthusiasm for the drugs results in some taking statins who don't need them, possibly leading to unnecessary side effects and risks. Others who have much to gain from lowering their cholesterol may rely on medication as a crutch, wrongly viewing it as an effortless alternative to lifestyle changes. Exercising, eating a healthful diet, and stopping smoking require more work than taking a statin, but the payoff to our health can be far greater. As Abramson put it, "Most heart disease results from the way we live our lives, and there's no magic pill to help us change that."

ECHO EFFECT

Of course, the NCEP doesn't act alone in spreading the word about statins, diet, or the dangers of high cholesterol. Anyone who spends at least a little time watching television regularly sees pharmaceutical ads touting the benefits of one cholesterol drug or another. Likewise, if you set foot in a grocery store even occasionally, you're sure to come across food labels that scream "no cholesterol" and products ranging from oatmeal to eggs that promise to help control your levels.

While the NCEP is not directly responsible for messages like these, it has created an environment that enables and encourages them. By raising the visibility of high cholesterol as a health risk and portraying it as a threat to everyone, the NCEP has paved the way for the burgeoning market of drugs, foods, dietary supplements, and other products that promise to protect us. The campaign's warnings are repeated and reinforced by manufacturers of these products, who have a financial incentive to stoke our concerns about cholesterol. The result is an echo effect that further amplifies the NCEP's message.

The NCEP's impact is also enhanced through its close collaboration with health groups such as the American Heart Association, the American College of Cardiology, and the American Medical Association. Messages for the public and recommendations for physicians are crafted in a way that secures the buy-in of these organizations, which then help spread the word. As the NCEP's director explains, such collaboration "has transformed what would otherwise be a federal project into a national program."

For example, the American Heart Association's cholesterol education program, called the Cholesterol Low Down, mirrors the NCEP in its mission of encouraging all Americans to "visit their doctors, learn their cholesterol numbers, and take action today to reduce their risk for cardiovascular disease." Like the NCEP, this campaign (which is sponsored by Pfizer, manufacturer of the statin Lipitor) issues population-wide warnings about high cholesterol, portraying it as a potentially deadly threat to everyone. Further, it points people to the NCEP's treatment targets and reiterates the NCEP's advice to first try lifestyle changes to lower cholesterol and then to consider medication if those changes don't work after three months.

Through its collaboration with and influence on groups such as the American Heart Association, the NCEP tries to ensure that "the messages of cholesterol education remain coherent and consistent." Having various health organizations sing the same tune can certainly be a good thing, but not if they're all off-key. By sticking to the NCEP's simplistic script, these groups engage in a form of educational collusion that leaves us less than fully enlightened about cholesterol. They also help minimize challenges to the NCEP's agenda, since we're less likely to question advice when it seems to be coming from everyone. But, as healthy skeptics, we should be asking questions. Just because multiple groups speak with one voice doesn't necessarily mean they're telling us the full truth, no matter how many there are or how respected they may be.

THE *REAL* CHOLESTEROL LOWDOWN

If the message you take away from this chapter is that you don't need to get your cholesterol checked or that you can just ignore a high number, that's not my intention. Yes, you should know your cholesterol numbers, as the NCEP urges; and, yes, you should discuss them with your doctor. But remember they're just one piece of a much larger puzzle. High cholesterol doesn't mean you're sick or necessarily need treatment, and a low or normal reading doesn't mean you're immune from heart disease. In short, resist the temptation to view your cholesterol score as a proxy for your overall heart health.

Whatever your cholesterol level, it's a good idea to exercise and to eat a healthful diet. If high cholesterol serves as a motivator, that's great. But if your levels fail to come down, avoid the common mistake of concluding that lifestyle measures aren't working and therefore can be abandoned. By sticking with the program, you'll be helping yourself in other ways that are perhaps even more important than lowering your cholesterol.

As for taking medication, it's a complex decision that involves more than just your cholesterol numbers. Among the questions to consider are these:

– What is my overall risk of heart disease?
– How much has the medication been proven to lower the risk of heart attacks, strokes, and death—in absolute terms, not relative ones—in someone of my gender and age, with my particular risk factors?
– What are the possible side effects, and how common are they in someone like me?
– What are the costs—for not only the medication but also tests to monitor safety?

When you encounter campaigns from the government and other entities about the hazards of high cholesterol or anything else, view them as you would any other marketing effort. Like enticements for cars or cruises, they may play up certain facts that don't apply to you and withhold others that do. In short, they don't always tell you everything you need to know to make an informed decision. It's up to you as a healthy skeptic to read the fine print before you buy.

TRUSTWORTHY SOURCES OF INFORMATION

Center for Medical Consumers (www.medicalconsumers.org). This independent group critically evaluates the evidence for medical and public health practices, including those related to high cholesterol.

The Statin Effects Study Web site (http://medicine.ucsd.edu/ses). Created by researchers at the University of California, San Diego, this site lays out the benefits and possible risks of statins in a clear and balanced way.

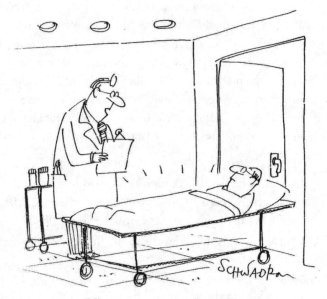

www.CartoonStock.com

"THE BODY SCAN, BONE SCAN, HEAD SCAN AND INTERNAL ORGAN SCAN WERE ALL NEGATIVE. THE BAD NEWS IS THAT YOU'RE RADIOACTIVE."

CHAPTER SIX: CELEBRITIES
GET TESTED!

I f you are an Oprah Winfrey fan (and even if you aren't), you know she's never been shy about opening up. She's shown anger, shed tears, and shared her childhood traumas and adult struggles in front of millions of viewers. In 2000, after years of baring her soul, the daytime talk diva took self-revelation to a new high when she decided to bare her liver, kidneys, and spleen as well.

In a now-famous episode of her popular TV program, Oprah underwent a full-body CT scan, which takes three-dimensional pictures of the inside of the body. Images of Oprah's innards were projected onto a large screen as the doctor who had performed the test, Harvey Eisenberg, discussed the results. Among other things, Oprah learned she had a small amount of plaque in her arteries and a bulging disc in her spine. Calling the test "miraculous," she told viewers it could "show dangerous diseases lurking in your lungs, in your liver, your arteries, even in your bones" and let doctors "possibly discover health problems before they become deadly."

What followed was a national frenzy over full-body scanning. Dr. Eisenberg's clinic was flooded with calls, as were imaging centers across the country. Within two years, dozens of new centers had opened to meet the growing demand. The test's hefty price tag of $1,000 or more—which insurance doesn't cover if you have no symptoms—wasn't enough to stop the worried well from clamoring to be scanned. As one observer noted,

Oprah's on-air test did for full-body scans what her reading club did for book sales.

But, unlike books, body scans aren't completely benign. Often they reveal apparent abnormalities when there's really nothing wrong, forcing people to undergo unnecessary follow-up tests that can be invasive and expensive. In addition, the dose of radiation they deliver can be high—as much as several hundred times that of a chest X-ray. As for the benefits, there are no studies showing that the scans save lives. But none of this seemed to matter much to Oprah. She saw her promotion of the scans as a public service, as "our step in getting people to think about prevention."

Oprah isn't the only celebrity-turned-health-promoter extolling the virtues of screening (defined as routine testing in people with no symptoms). Everyone from Rudy Giuliani to Rosie O'Donnell has taken on the cause of urging us to get regular tests of one kind or another. Whether it's a heart scan or a bone X-ray, a prostate test or a mammogram, the celebrities' messages are essentially the same: the earlier a condition is detected, the greater the chances of successfully treating it and heading off disability and death.

It's one of those often-repeated ideas that most of us take as a given. In one survey, nearly 87 percent of adults said that routine cancer screening is almost always a good idea, and three-quarters agreed that finding cancer early saves lives most or all of the time. For some conditions, such as cervical cancer and high blood pressure, substantial evidence exists that early detection can indeed be highly beneficial. But for other conditions, there's little or no evidence. Though it seems counterintuitive, routine testing and early intervention may not in fact always lead to better health or a longer life. And it's possible that screening may do harm by causing false alarms and unnecessary treatment.

Promotional efforts involving celebrities typically fail to convey this complexity. Instead, they usually tell us the test is "simple," playing up the benefits ("this test can save your life") or the consequences of not getting tested ("don't wait until it's too late"), without adequate attention to limitations and possible downsides. In many cases, these appeals are motivated by deeply emotional personal experiences such as the celebrity's own serious illness or the death of a loved one. In other cases, the celebrity is paid by drug or device manufacturers, which stand to benefit if more people get tested and treated. In still other instances, testing centers use a famous person's misfortune to scare us into getting screened. Whatever the particulars, the result is campaigns that are driven not by reason but by emotion or profit, neither of which should influence a decision as important as whether we get tested.

KATIE'S COLONOSCOPY CAMPAIGN

A slew of celebrities ranging from Magic Johnson to Michael J. Fox have helped raise awareness of various health issues, but perhaps none more so than Katie Couric. Since losing her husband, Jay Monahan, to colon cancer when he was 42, Couric has been a vocal advocate for early detection of the disease. When, as co-host of the *Today Show*, she promoted colon cancer screening by showing her own colonoscopy on the air, people signed up to be tested. In fact, researchers reported that colonoscopy rates rose by 20 percent or more after her on-air test, a phenomenon they dubbed the "Katie Couric Effect."

Colorectal cancer, which claims the lives of more than 50,000 Americans a year, is the second leading cause of cancer deaths. It's an example of a disease for which there's solid evidence that early detection does save lives. That's the conclusion of the U.S. Preventive Services Task Force (USPSTF), an independent panel of experts convened by the government to evaluate the research on screening and make recommendations. The panel suggests that everyone 50 and older be tested regularly, and various physicians' groups as well as the American Cancer Society agree. They all recommend one of several options: a fecal occult blood test (which measures blood in stool) every year; a sigmoidoscopy (which examines the lower part of the colon) every five years; or a colonoscopy (which allows doctors to see the entire colon) every 10 years. These groups also advocate initial screening at a younger age for those at higher risk of colon cancer because of a family history or other factors.

Age 50 has been designated as the time to begin testing, in part because the incidence of the disease increases substantially among people in their 50s and beyond. Before that, the risk is quite low in the general population—so low that to detect one cancer among people in their 40s, it's necessary to screen as many as 1,000 individuals. Consequently, the USPSTF and others do not recommend screening people under 50 who are not at increased risk. As the panel points out, the tests can have drawbacks: the fecal occult blood test can cause false alarms; sigmoidoscopy and colonoscopy can, in very rare instances, perforate the colon; and colonoscopy is done under anesthesia, which carries risks. For younger people, the benefits of screening may not outweigh these downsides.

Teaming up with the Centers for Disease Control and Prevention, Couric has appeared in public service announcements that target people 50 and older for testing. And during the many times she's talked about screening on the *Today Show* and elsewhere, she has specified that it's recommended for people in this age group. But not always. In an interview with *Good Housekeeping* magazine, Couric stated, "All the doctors I know—and I know a lot of them—say they had or will get a colonoscopy by their fortieth birthday. That ought to tell you something."

Such statements send a message at odds with science-based advice, as did Couric's on-air colonoscopy when she was in her 40s. As health journalism professor Gary Schwitzer observed: "She used her position as the co-host of a national television show to publicize her own choice to have a colonoscopy—even though there is no evidence-based guideline to support a colonoscopy in an otherwise healthy woman in her forties. Her husband's death from colon cancer had nothing to do with her risk."

The researchers who identified the Couric Effect noted a small decline in the mean age of people undergoing colonoscopies. This trend suggests that *Today Show* viewers, whose average age at the time was 47.5, may have followed the star's example and signed up for screening while in their 40s. Certainly, younger people can and do develop colon cancer, as evidenced by the tragic death of Couric's husband. And, undoubtedly, some people under 50 who got screened because of Couric ended up having cancer that was caught in the early, treatable stages. But the anecdotal experiences of individuals—who either didn't get tested and died or did get tested and lived—don't add up to proof that it's in the best interest of all 40-somethings to get tested.

Almost half of people 50 and older don't get screened, and the researchers who identified the Couric Effect suggest that celebrities such as Couric should target their messages to these individuals, for whom screening has been proven to be beneficial, rather than to younger people. But that's easier said than done. With the best of intentions, celebrities motivated by personal experience may be telling us what they believe in their hearts—not necessarily what science has determined to be true.

PUSHING FOR PSAS

Personal experience is also the impetus for celebrity campaigns promoting screening for prostate cancer. But, in this case, it's unclear whether routine testing is beneficial at *any* age. The tests for prostate cancer—the digital rectal exam (DRE) and the prostate-specific antigen (PSA) blood test—have long been controversial in the medical community. Both can detect cancers in early stages, but neither has been shown through randomized trials to save lives. The DRE misses many cancers, and the PSA may end up finding small tumors that are very slow growing and perhaps not life-threatening.

Prostate cancer is so common—after skin cancer, it's the most frequently diagnosed cancer in men—that if men live long enough, most end up developing it. For a small percentage of those who are diagnosed, the disease is deadly. (Though the percentage is low, the absolute number of deaths each year—more than 27,000—is relatively large.) For many more men, though, the condition is not fatal, and they die of something else. But because doctors can't predict whether a small, early-stage tumor will lie dormant or become lethal, most men opt for treatment, which can have fairly major complications, including impotence and incontinence. So while testing may in fact lead to life-saving treatment, it may also prompt remedies—and side effects—that are unnecessary.

Another drawback of the PSA is a fairly high false alarm rate. Various factors besides prostate cancer, including benign prostate enlargement, can cause PSA readings to be high. Men with abnormal levels typically must undergo repeat PSA tests and follow-up exams, including biopsies. And only about 25 to 30 percent of those who are biopsied because of a high PSA turn out to actually have cancer.

Because there's no conclusive evidence on whether the benefits out-weigh these downsides, the USPSTF recommends neither for nor against routine testing. Likewise, the CDC urges each man to discuss the pros and cons with his doctor and make his own decision. The Prostate Cancer Foundation, an advocacy group that raises money for research and provides information about the disease, similarly refrains from telling all men to be tested. On its Web site, the group lays out the pros and cons, advising that "because a decision of whether to be screened for prostate cancer is a per-sonal decision, it's important that each man talk with his doctor about whether prostate screening is right for him."

But at least one celebrity closely tied to the Prostate Cancer Foundation has a far less subtle message about screening. Former pro golfer Arnold Palmer, a prostate cancer survivor, is honorary chairman of a campaign called Arnie's Army Battles Prostate Cancer, which raises money for the Prostate Cancer Foundation. A vocal advocate of routine testing, Palmer says in a video message on his Web site, "Believe me, early detection is the key to beating prostate cancer. But we need to educate and encourage men to see their doctors and get tested." Pointing out that many men have told him they now get regular PSAs because of his recommendation, he added in an interview: "I know that there are also a lot of men who are NOT get-ting a regular PSA. I don't know how you can convince them that this sim-ple test might just save their life. I guess we just have to keep saying it over and over, stressing that this is something that is really very necessary."

Like Palmer, former New York City mayor Rudy Giuliani is a prostate cancer survivor and an ardent promoter of screening. But, unlike Palmer, Giuliani has been allied with a prostate cancer organization that shares his zeal for testing. The group, the National Prostate Cancer Coalition, pro-vides free screenings to men on mobile units that travel to communities across the country. As honorary chairman, Giuliani has advised: "If you're over 50 or in a high risk group, please get screened—now." This position mirrors the coalition's recommendation that all men begin annual PSA test-ing no later than age 50 and that African Americans and those at increased risk start at 40.

To spread its message, the group has also enlisted figures from Major League Baseball, including Hall of Fame shortstop Ozzie Smith and Chicago Cubs manager Lou Piniella. Both have served as spokesmen for a campaign called "Take a Swing against Prostate Cancer," intended to raise baseball fans' awareness of the risk of prostate cancer and the benefits of early detection. In interviews, Smith and Piniella have enthusiastically endorsed screening, noting that they get tested at least *twice* a year. Underlying their actions is the notion that the more often you get screened, the better your odds against prostate cancer—a belief that, while presumably sincere, is scientifically off base. No studies have ever shown this to be the case.

To back up its celebrities' assertions, the National Prostate Cancer Coalition points to five-year survival rates for prostate cancer, which have risen to 99 percent since the PSA came into widespread use. Though it sounds impressive, the statistic doesn't necessarily prove that the test saves lives. Because of increased screening, the number of men diagnosed with early, slow-growing prostate cancer has risen sharply, and nearly all of them live at least five years after diagnosis. But it's possible that many, if not most, would have lived five years anyway, and the statistic begs the question of whether early detection has allowed these men to live longer than they would have if their cancers had been found later or never at all.

In addition to trumpeting this somewhat misleading statistic, the coalition promotes its pro-screening agenda by attacking those who don't share its unbridled enthusiasm for routine testing. For example, in a letter to *Time*, the coalition's leader, Dr. Richard Atkins, went after the magazine's science editor for writing an article that presented both sides of the issue; Atkins argued that the article would give men "another excuse to avoid taking care of their health." Apparently, a one-sided celebrity anecdote would have been more to Atkins's liking. "Men over the age of 50 . . . should resolve to get tested annually," he wrote. "Senator Bob Dole, former New York Mayor Rudy Giuliani, retired General H. Norman Schwarzkopf, Michael Milken and Major League Baseball managers Joe Torre and Dusty Baker . . . would agree."

The coalition, which also works with NASCAR drivers and holds annual auctions of celebrity-designed beer bottles, relies heavily on famous people to raise awareness because the strategy works. In one survey, nearly two-thirds of men age 50 and older reported that they had seen or heard celebrities talking about PSA testing. About one-third of these men said a celebrity message had made them more likely to get screened. That translates potentially to millions of men who end up getting tested because of a celebrity endorsement. It would be fine if these men did so with a full understanding of both the benefits and the limits of testing. But because celebrities typically tell only half the story, their endorsements don't usually lead to fully informed decisions.

Dr. Gilbert Welch, part of the team that conducted the survey and a leading expert on cancer screening, warns that people should resist being swayed by stories, whether from friends, acquaintances, or celebrities. "The reason to get tested for cancer," he wrote in his book on the topic, *Should I Be Tested for Cancer?*, "is because it really saves lives (something that takes thousands of cases to prove), not because someone testifies that her own life was saved or that someone else's could have been."

BONE OF CONTENTION

Screening for osteoporosis also involves a host of unanswered questions, but that hasn't stopped celebrities from wholeheartedly endorsing it as well. Certainly, there's no question that osteoporosis, which makes bones more prone to fracture, can cause enormous suffering. Hip fractures, which occur mainly in the elderly, can rob people of their independence and even lead to death. Likewise, spinal fractures can cause deformity and pain. Though the condition can affect men, women are four times more likely to have it, and their risk rises after menopause. Screening can be useful for older women or those who are at high risk of fractures, but there's little evidence that testing all women when they hit menopause—the recommendation of many celebrities—will lead to fewer fractures decades down the road.

Screening tests for osteoporosis, which measure bone density, are noninvasive. The gold standard, known as dual-energy X-ray absorptiometry (DEXA), is performed on the hip or spine. With this or other tests, measurements can also be taken at the hand, wrist, forearm, or heel. Results are interpreted by comparing them to what would be expected in a healthy woman at about age 30, when bone mass is at its peak. The difference is called a T-score. A bone density that's 2.5 standard deviations or more below the ideal (a T-score of −2.5) indicates osteoporosis. Those whose T-scores fall between −1 and −2.5 are said to have osteopenia, or low bone mass.

Among those age 50 and older, nearly half of white women and more than one-fourth of black women fall into this gray zone of osteopenia. But it's unclear what, if anything, they should do, especially if they're in their 50s. Younger women are at relatively low risk of fractures, and having low bone density doesn't necessarily mean that someone will go on to develop full-blown osteoporosis. It's also worth noting that while lower bone density is associated with a greater chance of fractures, it's not the only contributor. Bone quality (which is different from density), weight, race, smoking, family history, muscle strength, physical activity, and likelihood of falling, among other things, are also important.

Yet in many cases, the results of a bone density screening test cause a woman to be labeled as having osteopenia—a condition that some cite as an example of disease-mongering. Frightened at the prospect of a hunched back and broken hips, women may automatically agree to take medication, perhaps unaware that the evidence is mixed as to whether it prevents fractures in those with osteopenia. And even if it does, the absolute decrease in risk is likely quite small. That has to be weighed against the possibility of side effects, which can range from rashes to rotting of the jaw. A woman in her 50s will probably have to take the medication for decades, and, for newer drugs, any long-term effects are unknown.

A panel of experts convened by the National Institutes of Health to review the science on osteoporosis concluded that the value of screening all women in their 50s was unproven. Similarly, the U.S. Preventive Services Task Force found insufficient evidence of a benefit to recommend routine testing for women under 60. Since the risk of fractures increases with age, USPSTF does suggest screening all women beginning at age 65 and a bit sooner, at 60, for those at greater risk because of low body weight or other factors.

If you listen to celebrities promoting osteoporosis screening, however, you get none of this nuance. Actress Rita Moreno, for example, has made the pronouncement that "bone density tests are the most important thing for a woman who is reaching or into menopause. It's vitally important that she get measured and find out what her bone health is about." The failure to get tested, she has said, is "absolutely criminal."

Similarly, actress and singer Debbie Reynolds—telling women emphatically that "you must take this test!"—went so far as to write a letter to advice columnist Ann Landers urging all postmenopausal women to talk to their doctors about getting tested. "Thank you for a letter that could improve the quality of life for millions of women," Landers responded. "You performed a valuable service by writing." Reynolds's "valuable service" also has included spreading highly misleading information like this: "If you test for it early enough, you need not get osteoporosis in the first place. It absolutely can be prevented."

At least Moreno and Reynolds, both over 65, are of the age at which routine screening is recommended by USPSTF—and so are many of their fans. The same can't be said of *Today Show* co-host Meredith Vieira, who at age 49 (before joining *Today*) headed a campaign urging all postmenopausal women to demand that their doctors perform bone density tests. "Tell them you really want to know your T-score," she urged, "because once you know your score, there is a lot that can be done."

In print and television interviews, Vieira spoke about her own bone density test, revealing that "I was surprised when I learned I had low bone mass." She reported that she didn't yet have osteoporosis—meaning that she had osteopenia—but noted, "If I continue to lose bone mass then I could develop it." As a result, she said, she was getting more calcium, doing more weight training, and—the clincher—"taking medication, as directed by my doctor."

It turns out that Vieira, Reynolds, and Moreno were paid spokespersons for initiatives funded by Merck, which manufactures the top-selling osteoporosis drug, Fosamax. Teaming up with the nonprofit National Osteoporosis Foundation (more on industry-funded nonprofit groups in the next chapter), the pharmaceutical giant has used these and other celebrities to front campaigns intended to get more people tested and thereby increase the number of potential customers (especially younger ones) for medications. Since Fosamax was approved by the Food and Drug Administration in 1995, Merck has made screening a centerpiece of its marketing efforts, promoting portable bone density testing machines for doctors' offices and investing in companies that make testing devices. It's no surprise, then, that the campaign for which Vieira was a spokesperson, called "Be Beautiful to the Bone: Know Yourself to a T," also involved free screening for women 50 and older at shopping centers around the country.

Press materials about the osteoporosis screening campaigns don't always disclose the company's sponsorship, and media outlets interviewing celebrity spokespersons don't always reveal that the stars are getting paid. When there is disclosure, it's sometimes only a fleeting, oblique reference. For example, when Meredith Vieira appeared on *Good Morning America* to talk about the importance of bone density testing and knowing your T-score (with no mention of who should be tested or the limitations of screening and early treatment), she was introduced only as a spokesperson for the National Osteoporosis Foundation. It wasn't until the end of the interview that co-host Diane Sawyer quickly added, "We wanna say the National Osteoporosis Foundation's 'Be Beautiful to the Bone: Know Yourself to a T' campaign is sponsored by Merck." While that brief statement perhaps satisfied *GMA*'s disclosure policy, it left viewers unaware that Vieira was a paid spokesperson and that Merck, her benefactor, makes an osteoporosis drug and has a financial incentive to get more people tested.

Limited as it is, such disclosure represents an improvement over previous practices. In 2002, Salon.com and the *New York Times* revealed that when stars such as Kathleen Turner and Lauren Bacall appeared on network morning programs to talk about health issues (and even to mention specific drugs), it was not disclosed that they were getting paid—in some cases as much as $1 million—by pharmaceutical companies.

Since having their journalistic lapses exposed, *GMA* and other members of the media have become a bit more cautious about celebrity health campaigns, but not enough, in many cases, to say no to them. According to public relations specialist Bob Brody, some outlets, such as *The View* on ABC as well as *Parade, People,* and *Prevention* magazines, "still love celebrity health campaigns no less than ever before." Brody is an executive in the health care practice of Ogilvy Public Relations Worldwide, which has been behind several dozen celebrity health campaigns, including the one in which Debbie Reynolds wrote to Ann Landers about bone density testing.

(Ogilvy boasts on its Web site that the letter reached 90 million readers.) Not surprisingly, Brody sees celebrity health campaigns as a good thing: "They educate. They leverage marquee value for a greater social good. They get results. . . . Patients initiate discussions with physicians, take diagnostic tests, and treatments are prescribed. Health is improved. Case closed."

But, in fact, the case is far from closed on whether celebrities perform a "greater social good" by telling all 50-something women to get screened for osteoporosis. Though PR professionals and celebrities who promote testing may sincerely believe that "health is improved" through their efforts, science suggests that the issue is far more complicated than that.

If testing reveals that you have osteoporosis and leads to drug treatment that heads off fractures, then your health may indeed be improved. The same is true if a bone density test motivates you to exercise more, stop smoking, and eat better. If, on the other hand, it causes you to become unduly alarmed and to take medication that subjects you to possible risks with little or no benefit, then you may end up worse off. Celebrities would perform a far greater public service if they at least made women aware of this complexity.

HEART-RENDING APPEALS

Sometimes celebrities can influence our decisions about testing without even intending to do so. For example, tests for heart disease known as cardiac CT scans are promoted through marketing campaigns that highlight the cardiac misfortunes of famous people—some of whom are dead. Sounding a "don't let this happen to you" alarm, the messages try to frighten us into getting tested. What they don't tell us is that, like other screening tests, cardiac CT scans have drawbacks that can outweigh the advantages for certain people.

The noninvasive tests, often referred to as electron beam tomography (EBT) or simply calcium scans, reveal whether blood vessels around the heart contain calcium, one of the components of artery-clogging plaque. In general, the more calcium there is, the greater the chances of coronary artery disease. But the test isn't foolproof. There can be considerable calcium buildup in people without heart disease, resulting in so-called false positive results that lead to unnecessary angiograms and other invasive and expensive follow-up tests. Conversely, it's possible to have plaque that doesn't contain calcium and therefore isn't detected by a CT scan.

USPSTF does not recommend the test for those who are at low risk of heart disease because the relatively high likelihood of false alarms outweighs any possible benefits. A different panel of experts who reviewed the evidence concluded that the test may be useful for certain people who have a couple of risk factors, such as smoking, high cholesterol, or high blood pressure. For such individuals, who are considered to be at intermediate risk, results from a calcium scan may help doctors better determine the chances of a future problem and the best approach to head it off. As for those who have heart disease or are at high risk for it, the test appears to provide little or no additional information to help tailor treatments.

Some clinics that offer the test haven't let such distinctions get in the way of their promotional efforts. Appealing to virtually all adults to get tested, they often rely on anecdotes, some about ordinary people who say they were saved by a scan and others about celebrities who supposedly could have been saved. One California testing center has included a page on its Web site with the heading "Could these deaths have been prevented?" There you can find obituaries of runners Jim Fixx and Brian Maxwell, actors John Ritter and John Spencer, and British rock singer Robert Palmer, all of whom died suddenly in their 50s, as well as baseball player Darryl Kile, who dropped dead at 33. They're all described as "people who might still be here today if only they had an EBT heart scan." The truth is that it's impossible to know whether a scan would have identified these individuals as high risk or, even if it had, whether taking action beyond what they were already doing would have prevented their deaths.

This clinic and others also cite the experience of former president Bill Clinton, who repeatedly passed treadmill stress tests but nevertheless ended up needing quadruple bypass surgery. In a press release, a Colorado clinic declared that Clinton's experience revealed the "limitations of stress tests and promise of EBT heart scans" and quoted a preventive cardiologist as saying that "there is no doubt that President Clinton would have been identified as high risk 10 years ago—if he had undergone calcium scan-

ning—and the odds are great that bypass surgery could have been avoided."
In fact, such a statement amounts to pure speculation, especially consider-
ing that the doctor who uttered it—a zealous promoter of cardiac CT
scans—wasn't involved in the former president's care.

When word got out about Bill Clinton's heart problems, many men
flocked to doctors and hospitals to have their hearts checked, a phenomenon dubbed the "Clinton Syndrome." Seeking to capitalize on this, some
clinics ran ads touting the test as key to avoiding Clinton's fate. For example, claiming that a CT scan would have "saved Mr. Clinton from a trip to
the operating room," one radio spot warned, "Don't be another statistic like
Bill. Insist upon the only proven test to detect early heart disease."

A radio ad for an Ohio clinic was more blunt, telling listeners, "Don't be
as dumb as Bill Clinton." Stating that the former president had "almost
died" and that a heart scan "could have easily discovered" his heart disease
"long before it was too late," the ad used fear to attract customers: "Two
hundred thousand Americans each year do find out too late," the narrator
ominously declared, "by experiencing sudden death from a heart attack
without prior symptoms, and two to three percent also die when having
bypass surgery." A cardiac CT scan, according to the ad, lets you "find out
if you're at risk when heart disease is easily corrected, or get the peace of
mind that you're OK." Missing from the ad was any mention of the limits
of calcium scans or who is and isn't a good candidate—essential elements
of a responsible message. Instead, everyone was urged to "do it now!"

Proponents often argue that the test can be a powerful motivator for
people to change their health habits. Though some research suggests otherwise (at least in relatively young, low-risk individuals), a high calcium
score may very well give you the incentive you need to eat better, exercise,
or stop smoking. If that's the case, the test may be well worth it. But a scan
may be counterproductive if it gives you false reassurance. Getting a clean
bill of health—which is what many test-takers seek—should not be taken
as a license to eat double cheeseburgers with abandon. At best, the test can
perhaps help predict your odds of having a heart attack. It can't confirm that
you're immune. Nor, despite what the ads imply, can it guarantee that you'll
escape the fate of Bill Clinton or other famous people.

RIGHT AND WRONG REASONS TO TEST

Five years after her famous full-body scan, Oprah was at it again, this time undergoing a CT angiogram, a highly advanced imaging test of the heart. Unlike a calcium scan, this test provides amazingly detailed 3-D pictures, showing arteries that are narrowed. Though no respected medical authorities recommend it as a screening tool for the general public, neither Oprah nor the two physicians on her program mentioned this. Instead, the show featured four viewers who "thought they could be at risk" for heart disease getting the test. Hailing it as a lifesaver, Oprah declared, "Don't be one of those crazy people who doesn't want the information, because information is power."

Oprah's aphorism is certainly true if you're engaged in car shopping or national security. But health is a different matter. Though information from screening tests can indeed be empowering and save your life, it can also be paralyzing and unnecessarily panic-inducing, and do little or nothing to benefit your health. It all depends on your particular situation and your personality. Before heeding appeals to get tested, it can be helpful to ask yourself a few questions.

- IS THERE SCIENTIFIC EVIDENCE OF A POSSIBLE BENEFIT FOR SOMEONE LIKE ME? To find out, the best place to start is USPSTF, which objectively reviews the evidence regarding numerous tests. (See Trustworthy Sources of Information at the end of this chapter.) You might also check with organizations such as the American Cancer Society or the American Heart Association. Keep in mind, however, that evidence-based recommendations involve benefits, harms, and costs for entire populations. What's true for large groups of people may or may not apply to you as an individual. Based on your own health history, risk, and preferences, it may be perfectly reasonable for you to get a test that's not endorsed by USPSTF or others. But their recommendations should at least be factored into your decision.

- HOW AM I LIKELY TO RESPOND TO AN ABNORMAL FINDING? Sometimes the best approach is to do nothing and to repeat the test later, especially if it has a high false positive rate. But if you're a worrier who can't stand uncertainty and will feel compelled to immediately undergo more testing or start treatment, you might want to think twice about being screened. Before getting tested, you need to make sure you're prepared for a false alarm and resolve to proceed calmly and cautiously if there's an abnormal finding.

– HOW AM I LIKELY TO RESPOND TO A NORMAL FINDING? Many people undergo screening tests for peace of mind, hoping to confirm that they don't have a particular condition and don't need to worry about it. But a screening test can miss things, and even if it's accurate, it can only reveal what your health status is at a given point; it cannot indicate what will occur months, years, or decades down the road. A test may therefore not be in your best interest if you let it lull you into a false sense of security and use it as an excuse to ignore measures like exercising or eating properly.

– WHAT KIND OF GAMBLER AM I? In the end, whether to have a test comes down to your tolerance for different types of risk. For the chance of heading off a serious or life-threatening illness, are you willing to accept the risk of a false alarm and the anxiety and possible harms that accompany it? Or are you willing to bet that you won't get the condition and, if you do, that early detection won't help? Either position can be perfectly rational depending on the test and your particular circumstances.

These are the factors that should determine whether testing is appropriate for you—not exhortations from or stories about famous people. It can be hard to resist such appeals, especially when they come from celebrities we trust and admire, who seem so sincere about trying to help us. There's no reason to doubt that they mean what they say, even if they're getting paid for giving advice. And screening clinic operators who market tests with celebrity stories by and large believe they're saving lives. But good intentions are not a sufficiently sound basis for health advice. Certainly, doing as they urge and getting screened for cancer, osteoporosis, heart disease, or any other condition may be a good decision, but only if you make it with full knowledge of the scientific uncertainties and potential drawbacks involved. By failing to give us this information, though, celebrities' well-intentioned efforts do us a disservice. And we do ourselves a disservice when we act without first asking questions.

TRUSTWORTHY SOURCES OF INFORMATION

The U.S. Preventive Services Task Force (www.ahcpr.gov/clinic/uspstfix .htm). This government-appointed panel of private-sector experts conducts impartial assessments of the scientific evidence for screening and other preventive services. On its Web page, you can find a list of tests and recommendations.

Should I Be Tested for Cancer? Maybe Not and Here's Why, by H. Gilbert Welch (Berkeley: University of California Press, 2004). This excellent guide to cancer screening clearly lays out the pros and cons of various tests and helps readers think through whether a particular test is right for them.

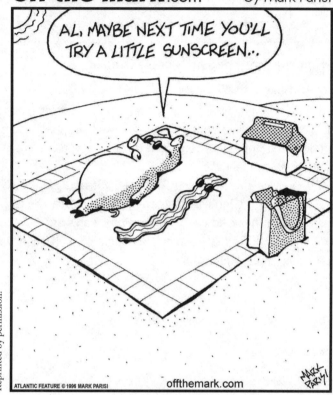

Reprinted by permission.

CHAPTER SEVEN: HEALTH GROUPS
WEAR SUNSCREEN!

Hardly anything is more wholesome than a community festival. Wherever it's held, you're likely to find all the familiar features, including lemonade stands, games for kids, and local artists displaying their crafts. If you've happened to visit festivals in cities such as Philadelphia, Atlanta, Cleveland, Denver, or Miami, you may have also seen something else: a booth for the "Families Play Safe in the Sun" campaign. The initiative is spearheaded by the Women's Dermatologic Society (WDS), an association of female skin doctors.

The campaign, whose mission is to "heighten sun safety awareness and practices among families," has traveled to events in 15 cities. At every stop, volunteer dermatologists give free skin cancer screenings and distribute sun safety educational materials to parents and their children. A key message is the importance of using sunscreen. On the campaign's Web site, you can find photos of smiling children being slathered with sunscreen, and the group's coloring contest for kids has awarded top prizes to drawings with captions such as "We all need sunscreen" and "Wear sunscreen!!" To drive the point home, volunteers frequently hand out as many as 15,000 free sunscreen samples to attendees—a fact that's played up in campaign press releases.

All this suggests that wearing sunscreen is one of the most important things—perhaps the most important—we can do to prevent skin cancer. It's a message we get from plenty of other sources as well, and we seem to be listening. When asked in one survey how they protected themselves from the sun, respondents were far more likely to list "apply sunscreen" than any other measure, including wearing a hat, extra clothing, or sunglasses.

This advice is so familiar—and so widely accepted—that it was even the subject of an imaginary graduation speech that was circulated on the Internet and later turned into a song. Written by *Chicago Tribune* columnist Mary Schmich (but falsely attributed to the late author Kurt Vonnegut), it began: "Wear sunscreen. If I could offer you only one tip for the future, sunscreen would be it. The long-term benefits of sunscreen have been proved by scientists, whereas the rest of my advice has no basis more reliable than my own meandering experience."

Sorry to say, it turns out that Schmich's one sure bet may not be so reliable either. While sunscreen can help protect us from sunburn and a less dangerous form of skin cancer, it has not been proven to guard against melanoma, the type that's deadly. Relying on sunscreen as a first line of defense—as educational messages and sunscreen giveaways may encourage us to do—can give us a false sense of security, leading us to wrongly believe we have carte blanche to bask in the sun. Research suggests that when we use sunscreen during activities such as sunbathing or swimming, we tend to stay in the sun longer than we would otherwise. Because sun exposure is linked to skin cancer, it's therefore possible that overreliance on sunscreen may wind up having the paradoxical effect of *increasing* the risk of certain skin cancers.

None of this is made clear to people stopping by a "Families Play Safe in the Sun" booth. Nor is it readily apparent that the sunscreen giveaway is anything more than just a friendly gesture by doctors. In reality, though, it's also a marketing opportunity for sunscreen makers, made possible by WDS. Like some other groups that aggressively push the importance of sunscreen, WDS has a cozy, symbiotic relationship with sunscreen makers. Sunscreen companies get implicit endorsements of their products from dermatologists, while WDS gets freebies to help endear itself to the public, along with financial support from several sunscreen manufacturers.

Other skin cancer awareness groups have even closer connections to the sunscreen industry. Whatever the exact relationship, when health groups are closely tied to sunscreen makers, they may not tell us all we need to know about the possible limitations of sunscreen.

As healthy skeptics, we need to keep in mind that even when the advice is as seemingly straightforward and innocuous as to wear sunscreen, and it's dispensed at events as innocent as community festivals, there can be hidden agendas. By remaining vigilant, we can avoid being misled by those who have an incentive to shade the truth.

SUNSCREEN SCIENCE

Since the early 1970s, sunscreen sales have soared roughly 30-fold, to more than $500 million annually. These figures suggest that the sunscreen message has largely sunk in. So does a visit to any beach on a summer day. Thirty or 40 years ago, it was common to see people sunbathing with suntan oils and reflectors intended to enhance the sun's effects. Today, in contrast, you'll see most people dutifully slathering themselves and their children with lotions that block the sun's rays.

Research shows that sunscreen does have definite benefits: it prevents sunburn and also helps guard against photoaging, the facial wrinkling, roughness, and discoloration associated with long-term sun exposure. In addition, we have evidence from various studies that sunscreen protects against a potentially disfiguring (and, in rare cases, deadly) but highly curable form of skin cancer known as squamous cell carcinoma.

The picture is cloudier when it comes to basal cell carcinoma, the least dangerous and most common type of skin cancer. (Together, basal and squamous cell cancers affect more than 1 million Americans annually.) There's little solid evidence that sunscreen reduces the risk of basal cell cancer. But because such lesions are so easily treated and so rarely fatal, the issue of prevention is far less urgent for basal cell cancer than for melanoma, which can spread rapidly to other parts of the body.

Every year, roughly 8,000 Americans die of melanoma. Caucasians are far more likely than other groups to develop the condition. Overall, the rate of new cases is about six times higher than it was 50 years ago, putting the disease among the 10 most common cancers. Though experts disagree on the reasons for this trend—some research suggests that it largely reflects greater vigilance by doctors—one thing is clear: increased sunscreen use has not led to a reduction in melanoma rates.

Conducting epidemiological research on sunscreen and melanoma is tricky: sunscreen products vary in effectiveness; people may not accurately remember how much they used; and factors such as skin type and time spent in the sun need to be taken into account. As a result of these challenges, studies have produced conflicting results. Some link sunscreen use to a decreased risk of melanoma, others link it to an increased risk, and still others detect no effect either way. Two analyses that pooled results from multiple epidemiological studies reached basically the same conclusion: using sunscreen neither decreases nor increases the risk of melanoma. Another review of sunscreen research, this one published in the *Canadian Medical Association Journal*, concluded that there's "no evidence of protective value" for sunscreen against melanoma and that "sunscreens should not be the first or sole agents used for skin cancer prevention." As one expert says, if sunscreens were regulated like prescription drugs, with manufacturers required to prove that their products prevent melanoma, "sunscreens would have failed the tests of efficacy during the approval procedure."

Those who promote sunscreen as a way to protect against melanoma frequently offer the following rationale: having more sunburns is linked to a higher risk of melanoma, and sunscreen prevents sunburns; therefore, sunscreen prevents melanoma. While the theory seems logical, it's not exactly bulletproof. For starters, research shows that when sunscreen-covered mice are exposed to UV light, they're protected against sunburn and other skin changes but not melanoma. Though human studies have found an association between sunburn and melanoma, the findings have been questioned, in part because people's recollections of their history of sunburn are often unreliable. Further, it's possible that sunburn is not itself a *cause* but rather a marker for a combination of other factors—fair skin, genetic susceptibility, and high sun exposure—that are actually responsible for the increased melanoma risk. If that's true, simply preventing sunburn may not necessarily head off melanoma.

Some researchers point out that studies to date have involved older, less effective sunscreens, and they believe that future studies on newer formulations will find a protective effect. Perhaps. Older sunscreens tended to block mainly ultraviolet B, or UVB, rays, which cause sunburn. Some newer sunscreens provide additional protection against UVA rays, which penetrate the skin more deeply than UVB rays and, according to research, may be an important contributor to melanoma. It's also possible, as some doctors suggest, that sunscreens would be shown effective if people applied them sufficiently and properly, which they often don't. Both explanations sound plausible enough, but the fact is that no one knows for certain whether they're true. They are unproven hypotheses intended to give credence to an unproven hypothesis.

That's not how science is supposed to work. Research always begins with the assumption of a "null hypothesis"—the idea that no association exists between two things (in this case, sunscreen and melanoma). Only by proving otherwise can we reasonably conclude that an association does exist. By first assuming that sunscreen prevents melanoma and then digging for supporting evidence and explanations as to why they can't find it, sunscreen proponents have turned science on its head. Their approach, more akin to religious faith than science, boils down to a belief that they're right, despite the lack of evidence, and a sense of optimism that eventually their views will be proven correct. Perhaps they will, but wishful thinking should never be a substitute for evidence-based advice, especially when people's lives are at stake.

Though scientists still don't fully understand the role of sun exposure in melanoma—the disease can occur on parts of the body where the sun rarely shines—the evidence strongly suggests that sunlight is a factor. The solution, then, is to reduce the amount of time people spend in the sun, especially if they're at increased risk, as evidenced by lots of moles, fair skin, and light-colored hair and eyes. Sunscreens may do the opposite by protecting users from sunburn and thus allowing them to stay out longer. Instead of being told what they want to hear—that it's possible to "play safe in the sun" by rubbing on some lotion—people should know the truth: that probably the best way to protect yourself is to cover up or go indoors.

GENEROUS BENEFACTORS

One of the most enthusiastic promoters of sunscreen is the Skin Cancer Foundation (SCF), a leading supplier of information about skin cancer prevention, detection, and treatment not only to the public but also to health professionals. The organization is frequently cited by the news media in stories about skin cancer. Like most other disease-focused groups, SCF is nonprofit, but its list of corporate benefactors reads like a who's who of sunscreen manufacturers. Companies such as Schering-Plough (maker of Coppertone), Sun Pharmaceuticals (Banana Boat), and Mary Kay (Sun Essentials) each pay an annual membership fee of $10,000 to sit on the group's Corporate Council. Many of these donors also supply additional funding for specific SCF initiatives. According to SCF, the contributions of council members provide "sustaining support for the Foundation's public awareness campaign and [help] disseminate the Foundation's vital message on a professional and consumer level."

If you visit the group's Web site, www.skincancer.org, you'll find plenty of information on sunscreen—how it works, which types to look for, how to apply it—but nothing about its effectiveness, or lack thereof, against melanoma. Though the group acknowledges that sunscreen is just one part of a complete protection plan, it portrays sunscreen as a first line of defense against all forms of skin cancer, equal in importance and effectiveness to other measures, such as covering up. And, in some cases, sunscreen is subtly singled out as first among equals. For example, in a section on its Web site titled "Year-Round Sun Protection," SCF lists these recommendations:

Use a sunscreen of 15 or higher whenever you spend time outdoors.
Cover up.
Seek the shade.
Never seek a tan.
Stay away from tanning parlors and artificial tanning devices.
Protect your children and teach them sun safety at an early age.

If the group wanted to be completely truthful, however, it would list sunscreen last, not first, making it clear that sunscreen has not been proven to reduce the risk of all forms of skin cancer and should therefore be a second line of defense.

Even more misleading is SCF's "seal of recommendation" program for sunscreens and other products that provide UV protection. Sunscreens that qualify can prominently display the SCF's "recommended" logo, giving consumers the false impression that the particular brand has been tested by SCF and proven to prevent skin cancer. In fact, the main criterion for displaying the seal is donating $10,000 to SCF to join the Corporate Council. Also, products must have a Sun Protection Factor (SPF)—an indicator of UVB protection only—of 15 or higher and must be backed by research involving at least 20 people. The laxness of these requirements means qualification is virtually automatic for most products whose manufacturers have shelled out the membership fee. Though the seal of recommendation appears to be a guarantee that products have been rigorously tested and shown to protect against skin cancer, it is actually a thank-you gift from SCF to its benefactors, who can and do cite the SCF's stamp of approval when touting the effectiveness of their products.

You can find the seal on sunscreens that promise "six-hour" or "all-day" protection but in fact supply no such thing. The effect is to reinforce the erroneous impression that it's okay to stay in the sun for extended periods. Similarly, the SCF seal is on products that claim to provide "broad-spectrum" protection against both UVA and UVB rays, even though studies show that many such sunscreens have only limited effectiveness against UVA. Further, some contain ingredients that break down in the sun. As of this writing, the Food and Drug Administration has no regulations in place regarding these issues (though new rules were proposed in August 2007), and the SCF seal has so far done nothing to fill the void. In essence, the program gives the SCF imprimatur to misleadingly labeled products in addition to reinforcing the widespread misperception that sunscreens are proven to protect against all forms of skin cancer.

Another seal you can find on certain Neutrogena sunscreens is that of the American Cancer Society. In return for a fee, the sunscreen manufacturer gets the right to use the logo of the nonprofit group. ACS describes this not as an endorsement but instead as part of a "cause marketing" relationship between the two organizations to promote skin cancer awareness.

One result of this arrangement is an edgy public service advertising campaign targeting young women. One of the ads, which has run in a number of women's magazines, shows a twenty-something woman holding a picture, with the headline "My sister accidentally killed herself. She died of skin cancer." At the bottom, it urges people to "make sun safety a way of life." What does that entail? First on the list that follows is to "use sunscreen," followed by "cover up" and "watch for skin changes." The ACS logo is featured, with no mention that Neutrogena paid for the ad.

In response to criticism of the campaign, the group's deputy chief medical officer, Dr. Len Lichtenfeld, wrote that "there is no conflict of interest" and that its message about skin cancer prevention "has not been influenced by an outside company." He urged others not to "assign or assume motives without an understanding of what was done and why."

Fair enough. But as long as ACS is so closely tied to Neutrogena—an arrangement that Lichtenfeld says gives his organization "the credibility and the visibility among publishers that we cannot obtain otherwise"—the group has a strong incentive to stick with the oversimplified message that sunscreen is an effective first line of defense against skin cancer. Adopting a more truthful and science-based stance—that consumers shouldn't count on sunscreen to prevent melanoma—would surely earn the disapproval of ACS's generous benefactor and likely mean the end of its marketing deal.

THE MASQUERADE BALL

In addition to funding health groups like SCF and WDS that promote sunscreen use, manufacturers and retailers sometimes create their own organizations whose ostensible purpose is to educate the public. For example, the Sun Safety Alliance is officially billed as a nonprofit organization whose aim is "to reduce the incidence of skin cancer by motivating people to actively adopt and practice safe sun behavior." The group's founders are the National Association of Chain Drug Stores (NACDS), whose members sell sunscreens, and Schering-Plough, maker of the top-selling sunscreen, Coppertone.

SSA is run out of the headquarters of NACDS by an association official, Phil Schneider. He is not a doctor or researcher, yet he has been quoted in SSA materials as an authority on skin cancer. Among his observations about the disease: "To stem this epidemic, it is critical that families adopt sun protection beyond spring and summer, to include year-round use of sunscreen, sun glasses, and hats."

Whenever the effectiveness of sunscreen is called into question, Schneider and the SSA are quick to come to its defense. For example, after the publication of a British study suggesting that sunscreens typically don't protect sufficiently against UVA rays and may give users a dangerous false sense of security, Schneider made a special effort to denounce the research. In a press release, he stated that "sunscreens are one of the most important weapons in the fight against sun-related skin cancer, *long recognized as the first line of defense*" (my italics). The release went on to misleadingly state that "most sunscreens protect against UVA" and to refer to "numerous studies" showing sunscreen to be a "necessary tool in the prevention of skin cancer."

When NACDS's then president Craig Fuller announced plans to form SSA at the association's 2002 annual meeting, he said SSA would include efforts to encourage consumers to purchase products that offer sun protection. By doing so, he explained, "the alliance will expand the base of future customers and appeal to the next generation of users of products or services made or sold by alliance allies, enhancing their sales."

SSA's mission to sell products is cleverly disguised, however. Instead of overtly pushing sunscreen, the group does so subtly, embedding its message in a broader effort to educate the public about sun protection and skin cancer. For example, SSA has declared the first week of every June to be "Sun Safety Week," the purpose of which is "to focus people's attention on the simple actions they can take to make sun safety a part of their everyday activities." The group has even persuaded Congress to pass a resolution that applauds SSA's efforts and "supports the goals and ideas of National Sun Safety Week."

Chief among those goals is boosting sunscreen use. To draw attention to the first annual Sun Safety Week in 2005, SSA commissioned a survey, which found that fewer people reported using sunscreen. SSA's press release, headlined "Sunscreen Use Down as Skin Cancer Rates Increase," began by describing sunscreen as a "primary protector against skin cancer." It went on to quote Brandi Donaldson, a melanoma survivor, who said that while growing up, "I spent a lot of time outdoors without any sunscreen"—a statement implying that her disease was caused by her failure to use sunscreen. "Now," she reported, "I don't think twice about applying sunscreen every morning before leaving the house—it's routine for me." The message was unmistakable: if you want to avoid melanoma, wear sunscreen.

Sunscreen also takes center stage in SSA's "Block the Sun, Not the Fun" educational program for second, third, and fourth graders. Among the lessons of this "sunlight and science literacy program" for classrooms is a demonstration on how sunscreen ingredients absorb, deflect, or scatter UV rays. Students are also instructed to visit Coppertone's Web site to check their city's UV index. Of the eight questions in the "Get Sun-Certified Quiz," which is supposed to test students' mastery of the material, five pertain to sunscreen. One, for example, asks:

Your mom wants to put some SPF 30 sunscreen on you. You say:

A. "No thanks, Mom!"

B. "Thanks, Mom! Now I don't have to worry for the rest of the day!"

C. "Thanks, Mom! Keep that close so we can reapply it later!"

In addition, the curriculum has included a letter-writing contest in which children offered their suggestions to the president on how to make their families or communities more sun safe. One of the winners was second grader Jacob Mendez, with the suggestion to "install a pump full of sunscreen at every playground and at swimming pools, near the restrooms or water fountains." For his idea, Jacob won a $750 savings bond, his school won a $100 gift certificate and a video microscope, and the SSA won over what it hopes will be another lifelong sunscreen customer.

Yet another tactic employed by SSA has been to create an offshoot organization called Mothers and Others against Skin Cancer. Former first lady Barbara Bush serves as its honorary chair. In a written statement posted on SSA's Web site, she hails the "commitment to building a national grassroots movement of 'mothers and others' who will take an active role in promoting simple, year-round sun safety practices." The idea that this effort is "grassroots," however, is nonsense. It's a classic example of a phenomenon sometimes called "astroturfing"—the creation of fake grassroots campaigns. While these efforts purport to be driven by ordinary people who are passionate about a cause such as preventing skin cancer, they're actually created and run by corporate entities, which use them as a way to advance their own agendas.

The goal of Mothers and Others is to sign up 1 million people who want to "show that they are concerned about children's health and preventing skin cancer." As an inducement, SSA has offered the chance to win a four-day, all-expense-paid trip to a Disney theme park. On its Web site, it also tells prospective enrollees they'll receive coupons for sunscreens and other sun-related products. Through this "grassroots" effort, SSA can encourage even more people to buy and use lots of sunscreen.

SSA also manages to propagandize through the news media without appearing to do so. In a 2003 segment on the *Today Show* announcing the group's launch, co-host Katie Couric began by talking about SSA's mission of educating children and families about sun protection. Referring to the group as a "new nonprofit organization," she did not mention its corporate parents. Joining her was Karen Graham, who had lost her 22-year-old son to melanoma. SSA promotes the efforts of Ms. Graham and the foundation she started, which successfully pushed for legislation in California allowing children to use sunscreen at school without a doctor's note. (Surprisingly, not all schools permit this.) After telling the moving story of her son's struggle with melanoma, she said that she was keeping the promise she had made to her dying son to "beat this disease" by working with SSA to pass similar legislation in every state in the country.

Also appearing in the segment was Dr. Jeff Ashley, a board member of SSA. He answered questions about how to apply sunscreen properly without offering even a hint of uncertainty about its effectiveness. During the course of their conversation, Couric stated that "regular use of a sun block . . . can lower the risk of certain types of skin cancer by up to 78 percent, which is phenomenal"—a finding repeatedly cited by SSA that is derived from mathematical models, not direct evidence. Dr. Ashley never bothered to mention that this statistic did not apply to melanoma, the type of cancer that had claimed Karen Graham's son.

A product promotion campaign ingeniously framed as public education had managed to use Couric as its pitchwoman. And if she didn't catch on to what was really happening—after all, the combination of a determined mother, an earnest doctor, and a public-spirited nonprofit group is hardly eyebrow-raising stuff—then surely her viewers didn't either.

THE OTHER SIDE OF THE SUN

One of the few criticisms of SSA has come from the indoor tanning industry. Wolff System Technology, the leading manufacturer of lamps for tanning beds, has called it a "self-serving advocacy group" that is "masquerading as an objective professional association." Among other things, Wolff objects to SSA's refusal to acknowledge the possibility that exposure to UV light may in fact be beneficial. Of course, Wolff's position is self-serving, too: it promotes indoor tanning, which has been linked to a higher risk of melanoma. However, the company makes a somewhat valid point when it comes to the possible benefits of sunlight.

Some research has linked greater sun exposure to lower incidence and mortality rates for various cancers, including prostate, breast, and colon cancer as well as non-Hodgkin's lymphoma. Studies have also found higher sun exposure during childhood and adolescence to be associated with a lower risk of multiple sclerosis. The skin makes vitamin D from sunlight, and researchers theorize that getting too little sun can cause a vitamin D deficiency and thereby lead to an increased risk of cancer and other conditions.

Among those making this case is the nonprofit UV Foundation, whose stated goals are to "increase the public awareness of the biologic effects of ultraviolet light" and create "a better public understanding of the calculus between benefits and risks of UV light." But a balanced approach is not what you actually get from the foundation. Serving as sunlight's chief cheerleader, it focuses entirely on the positive effects and exaggerates the strength of the evidence.

If you dig below the surface a bit, you'll find that the UV Foundation's financial backers are the Indoor Tanning Association (whose Web site includes a link to the UV Foundation's site) and several companies from the indoor tanning industry. Clearly, they have a financial incentive to spread the word that UV exposure is good for us, and this supposedly objective scientific organization offers them a credible vehicle for doing so. As it turns out, Wolff's characterization of SSA as a "self-serving advocacy group" is an equally apt description of the foundation tied to the company's own industry.

INCOMPLETE ADVICE

When rival groups dedicated to public education make competing claims, and both are advancing the interests of their respective benefactors, whom and what are we supposed to believe? In this case, you'd think that a group such as the American Academy of Dermatology (AAD), whose existence doesn't depend on the largesse of either industry, would be a source for complete and honest information. Unfortunately, that's not so.

To be sure, the group provides more balanced information about sunscreen than does the Skin Cancer Foundation or the Sun Safety Alliance. Says an official of the AAD: "People shouldn't feel they can stay in the sun for extended periods of time just because they are wearing sunscreen." But the academy supports the efforts of SSA—it even serves on the group's advisory board (as does the Skin Cancer Foundation)—and in its public education materials, you won't find any mention of the scientific uncertainty regarding sunscreen's effectiveness against melanoma.

An episode involving Dr. Marianne Berwick, an epidemiologist at the University of New Mexico, is telling. In 1998, Berwick made a presentation at a scientific meeting in which she reviewed 10 studies on sunscreen and melanoma, including one she had conducted. Her conclusion: "We don't really know whether sunscreens prevent skin cancer."

That honest admission, uttered at a gathering covered by journalists, made headlines across the country. The AAD, alarmed at the message this was sending, issued a press release denouncing Berwick's analysis as "misleading and confusing." In it, the group's president-elect called Berwick's assertions "a potential setback to over 20 years of sun safety public education" and ominously warned that "if only 10% of Americans who now use sunscreen stop, the seeds will be sown for an additional one million new cases of skin cancer in the next 10 years."

In interviews with the press, another AAD official attacked Berwick personally, deriding her as a "numbers cruncher, not a doctor." Never mind that Berwick had published numerous papers on melanoma. The group also sent a letter to Berwick, which was copied to her then employer, Memorial Sloan-Kettering, as well as to the American Medical Association, the American Cancer Society, the Centers for Disease Control and Prevention, the FDA, and major media outlets. Scolding her for causing "widespread public confusion" and "immeasurable harm," it demanded that she publicly "correct" her previous statements and "cease misleading comments in public interviews." Otherwise, said the AAD, her remarks could lead millions of people "to ignore sunscreens, get sunburned and subsequently develop skin cancers."

Underlying this overwrought reaction is an apparent belief that members of the public, like children, need clear, simple, unambiguous directions they can easily understand. Admit any doubt, the thinking goes, and they'll stop listening and obeying. Berwick's "crime" was to put greater faith in people, understanding that they deserve—and can handle—the full truth. While the AAD fretted over the possible fallout from Berwick's honesty, it seemed to disregard the potentially more serious consequences of its oversimplified message that sunscreen prevents skin cancer.

The AAD's paternalistic approach toward the public—best summed up as "keep it simple; they're stupid"—is perhaps also responsible for its less than complete information on sunlight and vitamin D. Trying to counter the one-sided, pro-sunlight message of the UV Foundation and others, the AAD takes an equally unbalanced stance in the opposite direction. For example, in a document titled "Research Shines Dangerous Truth on Sun Exposure and Vitamin D," the AAD essentially ignores emerging evidence linking sun exposure to health benefits. Instead, it warns about the hazards of the sun and tells people they can get adequate vitamin D through food and supplements.

Conspicuously absent from this advice are the crucial points that supplements have their own possible drawbacks, that it isn't always easy or even possible to get enough vitamin D through food, and that sunlight is by far the most efficient source of vitamin D. Depending on the season, the time of day, and where you live, as well as your skin type, brief sun exposure can provide thousands of international units (IUs) of the vitamin. In contrast, a 4-ounce piece of salmon delivers about 400 IUs, and a glass of milk has 100. The recommended daily level for adults is 200 to 600 IUs, depending on your age, and some nutrition researchers believe that it should be considerably higher.

Whether the issue is sunlight and health or sunscreen and melanoma, the American Academy of Dermatology selectively tells us what it thinks we need to know. Fearing that fully exposing all the facts may prompt some people to overexpose themselves to the sun, it omits certain key details and overstates—or understates—the strength of the evidence. The result is that we're left in the dark.

SHEDDING LIGHT

We should beware of any group, whether industry funded or not, that speaks with absolute certainty about this subject. Scientific knowledge regarding sunscreen and the effects of sunlight is still evolving. Those who are leveling with us will admit this reality, distinguishing between what's proven and what's not. Their list of dos, don'ts, and maybes might look something like this:

- The most effective way to protect yourself is to minimize your time in the sun, especially at peak hours. When you're out, wear a wide-brimmed hat and sunglasses, and seek the shade. If possible, cover up with clothing that's dark colored, made of tightly woven fabric, or specially treated to block UV radiation.

- Sunscreens do guard against sunburn, photoaging, and squamous cell cancer. It's possible that they also reduce the risk of basal cell cancer and melanoma, but the evidence for this is weak.

- Given their proven and possible benefits, it certainly makes sense to use sunscreens. But don't regard them as a first line of defense against melanoma or a license to spend long periods of time in the sun.
- For sunscreen to be effective, it needs to be applied copiously and reapplied often. Disregard labels such as "waterproof" and "all-day protection." Choose products with an SPF of 15 or higher, and look for ingredients such as zinc oxide, titanium dioxide, avobenzone, or Mexoryl SX, which provide UVA protection.
- It's possible that exposing your arms and legs to the sun (without sunscreen) for 10 minutes a day, two or three times a week, may be beneficial, depending on where you live and what season it is. The evidence for this is still emerging, however, and it doesn't mean sunbathing is safe.

Whether the subject is sunscreen or anything else, don't assume that a health group is completely trustworthy just because it's nonprofit and devoted to public education. Check out its Web site to find out who its financial backers are, how closely they're affiliated with the group, and what they potentially have to gain if information is spun a particular way. If the organization keeps its list of supporters a secret, consider it a red flag.

At the same time, don't assume that a group is deceitful just because it gets funding from industry. Many health organizations receive corporate dollars without sacrificing their honesty and independence. The question is whether the group's agenda and information are geared toward furthering the funder's financial interests. That's not always easy to answer, of course. But, as healthy skeptics, we need to keep asking.

TRUSTWORTHY SOURCES OF INFORMATION

The British Columbia Centre for Disease Control (www.bccdc.org/content.php?item=45). This group's Web site provides an excellent overview of the effects of UV exposure, laying out the facts about sunscreen and other protective measures in a thorough and balanced way.

The Integrity in Science Database (http://cspinet.org/integrity/
nonprofits/index.html). Offered by the Center for Science in the
Public Interest, this database identifies corporate donors who support nonprofit groups. It also contains information regarding industry support for scientists and universities.

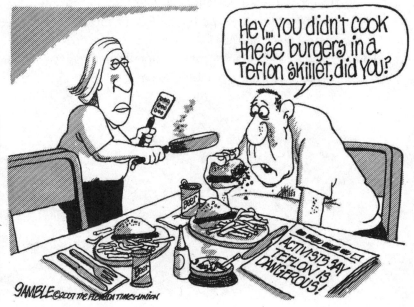

Ed Gamble © 2007 The Florida Times-Union

CHAPTER EIGHT: CONSUMER ACTIVISTS
BEWARE OF CHEMICALS!

I f there's a single fruit people most associate with wellness, it's the apple. Everyone has heard, after all, that one a day keeps the doctor away. The fruit's wholesome image took a nosedive in the spring of 1989, however, thanks to the work of an environmental activist group and the news media. In a now infamous episode, this perennial symbol of health was temporarily tagged with a skull and crossbones.

For years, the group, the Natural Resources Defense Council (NRDC), had been pushing for the ban of a chemical called Alar, which was sprayed on apples to regulate their growth. Studies in lab animals suggested that a by-product of Alar, known as UDMH, caused cancer. But the doses at which this occurred were massive—as high as 266,000 times the amount to which humans might be exposed—making the relevance of the research questionable.

To raise awareness of Alar and other agricultural chemicals, NRDC issued a study in 1989 focusing on children, who, it said, were especially vulnerable because they consume more fruit for their size than adults. Titled "Intolerable Risk: Pesticides in Our Children's Food," the report singled out UDMH as posing the "greatest cancer risk" among the 23 chemicals identified. Extrapolating from the dubious animal data and using equally questionable estimates of children's apple consumption, the study calculated that Alar was causing cancer in thousands of preschoolers. These risk levels, according to NRDC, were hundreds of times higher than those considered acceptable by the Environmental Protection Agency (EPA).

The controversial report was never subjected to peer review or published in a scientific journal. Instead, it was released directly to the news media, with CBS's *60 Minutes* given exclusive first rights. Calling the report "the most careful study yet," correspondent Ed Bradley told the program's 40 million viewers that Alar was "the most potent cancer-causing agent in our food supply."

The *60 Minutes* report was just the first salvo in a carefully orchestrated media blitz by NRDC. The next day, 13 news conferences were held across the country, followed a week later by an event at which actress Meryl Streep announced the formation of an NRDC "astroturf" group called Mothers and Others for Pesticide Limits. Every television program from *Donahue* to the *MacNeil/Lehrer NewsHour* jumped on the story, as did countless newspapers and magazines. *Time* and *Newsweek* devoted their covers to it.

The result was public panic. People threw away their apples and dumped out their apple juice. Supermarkets removed the fruit from shelves, and schools banned it from cafeterias. Sales of apples and apple juice tumbled, costing the apple industry hundreds of millions of dollars and forcing some growers out of business.

Trying to quell the furor, three government agencies—the Food and Drug Administration, the EPA, and the U.S. Department of Agriculture— released a joint statement that included the following points:

The data used by NRDC were invalid, and the report's risk estimates were inflated.

The risk posed by Alar was "not of sufficient certainty and magnitude" to require an immediate ban.

It was safe for children and adults to eat apples and other fruit.

But the reassurance was of little use. The scare subsided only after Alar's manufacturer, Uniroyal Chemical, decided in June 1989 to stop selling the product for use on food. NRDC had achieved its goal of getting rid of the chemical.

The organization also had another reason to celebrate: thanks to all the publicity, it was raking in new members and contributions. The man deserving much of the credit was David Fenton, founder of the public relations firm Fenton Communications, which NRDC had hired to mastermind the marketing around the release of its report. In a memo, Fenton described his objective this way: "to create so many repetitions of NRDC's message that average American consumers . . . could not avoid hearing it. . . . The idea was for the 'story' to achieve a life of its own, and continue for weeks and months to affect policy and consumer habits." He called the campaign "a model for other non-profit organizations."

Today, various "watchdog" public interest groups routinely employ similar tactics to raise awareness of other chemicals they allege are harmful. As with Alar, however, the science behind their claims is often far less solid than their marketing efforts lead us to believe. Seeking attention and financial support, and perhaps driven by missionary zeal, they may be strongly motivated to overstate their case.

Simply because they're looking out for our welfare doesn't necessarily mean that public interest groups always tell us the truth. Rather than helping us, they can sometimes cause harm by frightening us unnecessarily and diverting our attention from risks that are far more important. As healthy skeptics, we need to apply the same scrutiny to their advice as we give to that from industry-funded groups or anyone else.

LETHAL LIPSTICK?

A technique used with increasing frequency by consumer activists is to run eye-grabbing ads in high-profile publications. "Taking out an ad in a prestigious newspaper makes an organization look legitimate," explains activist leader Charlotte Brody. "The fact that you have the money to run the ads makes the world take you more seriously."

Brody has been involved with the Campaign for Safe Cosmetics, a coalition of health, women's, and environmental organizations that in recent years has relied heavily on advertising to get its message across. Appearing in the *New York Times*, *USA Today*, and *Ms.* magazine, among other places, the ads have sounded scary warnings about the dangers of certain substances, known as phthalates, that are found in a wide array of beauty products. Fenton Communications, the firm responsible for the Alar scare, developed some of the advertising, relying on its old trick of stirring up fear to advance its clients' causes.

Phthalates serve a variety of functions in beauty products, such as making fragrances last longer and preventing nail polish from chipping. In one analysis, FDA scientists found the chemicals in two-thirds of the cosmetic products they tested, including skin lotion, deodorant, body wash, shampoo, and hair spray.

Several of the ads, showing a large photo of a young girl applying lipstick, prominently displayed the line "Putting on makeup shouldn't be like playing with matches." One went on to state: "When it comes to cosmetics, we shouldn't be forced to choose between health and beauty. Personal care products should be free of chemicals linked to cancer and birth defects." Another showed a pregnant woman sniffing perfume, with text that read, "Sexy for her. For baby, it could really be poison." This ad and several others warned that phthalates "have been shown to damage the lungs, liver and kidneys, and to harm the developing testes of offspring. These results come from animal tests which, according to government scientists, are relevant to predicting health impacts in humans."

Well, not quite. While it's true that phthalates have been found to cause damage in rodents, the doses at which effects occurred far exceed levels to which humans are typically exposed. According to a report by the Centers for Disease Control and Prevention, that difference and other factors "make it difficult to translate the effects observed in animals to health effects in people."

The ad showing the perfume-sniffing pregnant woman cautioned that "toxic chemicals linked to birth defects are being found at alarming levels in women of childbearing age." Again, the rhetoric doesn't quite match reality. A CDC study analyzing 289 human urine samples for phthalate metabolites (or breakdown products) did indeed find higher phthalate concentrations among women of childbearing age. But follow-up research by the CDC involving a much larger sample showed levels in younger women to be the same as those in other women.

Some human research has linked higher levels of certain phthalate metabolites with premature breast development in young girls and sperm-related problems in men. But the studies are too small and preliminary to permit any definitive conclusions. In another preliminary study, pregnant women with greater phthalate concentrations in their urine were more likely to bear sons with a shorter than expected distance between the anus and the base of the penis (known as anogenital distance, or AGD). All the infants studied appeared normal, however, and it's not clear what, if any, adverse effects might be associated with these shorter AGDs.

Even if our everyday contact with phthalates does pose a health risk, it's misleading to single out cosmetics as the main culprit. The chemicals are found in hundreds of products, ranging from vinyl flooring to toys, and food (especially meat and fish) is thought to be a major source of exposure in adults. As for the role of beauty products, FDA scientists have found that some of those mentioned in the ad campaign, including soaps, shampoos, and conditioners, result in "very low" phthalate exposure because they're typically washed off the skin soon after application. Likewise, exposure from nail polish—another prime target—is low because the polish quickly hardens after being applied, limiting how much phthalate is absorbed.

Overall, the FDA's position is that it "does not have compelling evidence that phthalates, as used in cosmetics, pose a safety risk." An expert panel of the Cosmetic Ingredient Review, which is industry funded but conducts independent research and publishes findings in peer-reviewed journals, has likewise concluded that even when multiple cosmetic products are used, phthalate exposure levels are well below those found to be toxic to animals.

At the same time, the possibility of harm can't be ruled out, and more research is certainly warranted to follow up on preliminary studies that suggest possible adverse effects. But that's a far cry from asserting, as the ads do, that cosmetics are "poison" and "toxic."

One of the main purposes of the ads run by the Campaign for Safe Cosmetics has been to create public alarm and outrage sufficient to pressure manufacturers to remove phthalates and other allegedly harmful chemicals from their products. Says one ad: "We believe that every consumer— indeed, anyone who cares about the health of future generations—should

demand action from companies." In some cases, the ads have cited manufacturers by name, chastising them for not acceding to the Campaign's
demands. For example, one denounced OPI Products for making "some of
the world's most toxic nail products" and revealed that the company had
refused requests to make its products phthalate-free. "We know because we
asked their top executives in person," said the ad, which exhorted consumers to "Help Us Give OPI a Makeover." Eventually, the company
agreed to reformulate its products.

Some of the ads have also included a political call to action, urging the
public to demand stricter oversight by the FDA, which is responsible for
regulating the safety of cosmetics. "Tell the FDA that chemicals should not
be allowed in cosmetics products," urged one, "without first being assessed
for health and safety."

Reasonable people can disagree about how far society should go with the
so-called precautionary principle—the idea of better safe than sorry—and
how much evidence is sufficient to justify removing phthalates from beauty
products. The European Union has chosen to ban the use of certain phthalates because of its policy of acting against chemicals if even a suspicion of
harm exists. And the state of California requires cosmetics manufacturers to
report whether their products contain certain substances—including
phthalates—that are merely suspected of causing cancer or reproductive
problems.

The activist groups that are part of the Campaign believe in erring on
the side of safety, and they have every right to try to influence corporate and
government decision makers to adopt this viewpoint. The problem is their
tactic of trying to frighten and manipulate us by portraying phthalates as a
serious, well-established threat to each of us individually. If they were truly
acting in the public interest, they would address this as a societal safety
issue, not a personal one, and direct their appeals to corporate and public
officials without trying to whip up public hysteria. For consumers, they
would lay out the science in an honest and balanced way, acknowledging
that the risks are still unproven and that, if they do exist, they are likely very
small for individuals relative to other health threats. We would then have
the information required for making rational personal decisions about how
much energy and attention to devote to this theoretical threat.

When, instead of educating us with facts, activists try to influence us with alarmist advertising campaigns that warn us about being "poisoned" by shampoo or perfume, we may make irrational decisions because our actions are driven largely by fear. They win attention for their cause, but we lose our way in our quest for health.

SLIPPERY JOURNALISM

Activists frequently communicate through the news media, which tend to give the groups sympathetic treatment as heroes in a narrative of good versus evil. The familiar storyline goes something like this: the villain (usually a profit-crazed corporation) is somehow putting our health at risk without our knowledge, and the heroes (the activists) are coming to our rescue by exposing this nefarious behavior and loudly demanding that it cease. Rarely is there much journalistic scrutiny of the heroes' credibility or motives. Nor is there any perspective from independent experts. In the name of "balance," the villains get a chance to refute the heroes' claims, but their statements are often relayed by reporters with raised eyebrows. It's no surprise, then, why activists are so fond of working with the media and so reliant on them for advancing their agendas.

Consider the case of Teflon, the nonstick coating on cooking surfaces. Its production involves a chemical called perfluorooctanoic acid (PFOA), also known as C8. Countless other products in a wide array of industries are also manufactured using PFOA, including stain-resistant coatings on carpet and clothing, grease-absorbing surfaces on food packaging, and fire-resistant insulation on wire and cabling. Though the chemical is produced as an intermediate step during the manufacturing process, the final products typically contain, at most, only tiny amounts of it.

For years, activists have been pushing for a ban on PFOA, citing studies in rodents showing that it causes cancer and birth defects. They also point out that the man-made chemical is everywhere. For reasons that aren't fully understood, traces of it are found in everything from fish to polar bears. Virtually all Americans have PFOA in their blood. However, the levels tend to be extremely low—about five parts per billion. That's up to 25,000 times less than the amount demonstrated to cause harm in lab animals. Because of the difficulty of extrapolating the animal data to people—and the lack of evidence of serious harm to humans—scientists aren't sure whether our exposure to the chemical poses a health risk.

Acknowledging that "the science is still coming in," the EPA neverthe-less has decided to do what it calls "the right thing . . . for our environment and our health." Acting on the precautionary principle, it has urged indus-try to work toward eliminating PFOA from manufacturing emissions and products by 2015. Eight major companies, including Teflon's manufacturer, DuPont, have voluntarily agreed to comply.

As for what the public should do, the EPA states that currently it "does not believe there is any reason for consumers to stop using any consumer or industrial related products because of concerns about PFOA." It further points out that there's no indication we're being exposed to PFOA through Teflon cookware.

The Environmental Working Group (EWG), whose stated aim is to "expose threats to your health and the environment," has for years por-trayed Teflon as a serious health hazard and called for a ban on PFOA. It has also aggressively gone after DuPont, accusing the company of "pollut-ing drinking water and newborn babies with an indestructible chemical [PFOA] that causes cancer, birth defects, and other serious health problems in animals" and of trying to cover it up.

In a 2003 report titled "Canaries in the Kitchen: Teflon Toxicosis," EWG warned that, when heated, Teflon can break down and release toxic gases that kill birds and cause flulike symptoms in people. According to tests commissioned by EWG, such temperatures can easily be reached in just a few minutes during normal cooking. Taking aim at the group's archenemy DuPont, the report claimed that the company had misled consumers about these dangers. EWG petitioned the Consumer Product Safety Commis-sion (CPSC) to require that nonstick cookware carry a warning label, and it advised consumers to "phase out the use of Teflon or non-stick cookware in your home."

In fact, the threat to birds has been known for years, and DuPont read-ily acknowledges it. On the Teflon Web site, the company describes the problem and advises bird owners to take precautions such as keeping their pets out of the kitchen while cooking, never preheating cookware on high heat, and always making sure the kitchen is properly ventilated.

As for threats to people, it has also long been known that at very high temperatures—well beyond 500 degrees—Teflon can break down and cause flulike symptoms that go away within 24 to 48 hours. But there's no direct evidence for EWG's assertion that normal cooking temperatures have this or other adverse effects, nor is it necessarily true that what harms birds also harms people. Consequently, the CPSC rejected EWG's petition to require warning labels.

If you had happened to see a report about Teflon on ABC's *20/20* in November 2003, however, you wouldn't have learned about any of this. Instead, chief investigative reporter Brian Ross directed his incredulity entirely at DuPont, letting EWG's unproven assertions go largely unchallenged.

The report began with the story of Bucky Bailey, who was born with one nostril and a deformed eye. His mother, Sue, blamed her workplace, a DuPont plant in West Virginia where Teflon was made. Ross failed to mention that this was just an opinion; there was no research linking such problems to working in the plant.

After presenting this incriminating anecdote, the segment described how PFOA might be harming us all. Jane Houlihan, EWG's vice president for research, who appeared several times during the story, warned that Teflon and other stain-resistant chemicals "can absorb directly through the skin." Ross let this scary and misleading statement stand without elaboration or evidence. But when Uma Chowdhry, a senior official at DuPont, made a scientifically valid point—that PFOA's ubiquity doesn't necessarily mean it's harmful—the reporter's demeanor shifted from supine to sarcastic:

> *Chowdhry:* "Everyone has it."
> *Ross:* "It's in my blood, your blood?"
> *Chowdhry:* "We do not believe there are any adverse health effects."
> *Ross:* "Is it a good thing to have it in your blood?"

That exchange was followed by another unchallenged exaggeration from Houlihan: that levels in people are "too close to the levels that harm lab animals." Equally misleading was Ross's reference to "worrisome laboratory studies" of PFOA. Worrisome in what way? Ross failed to explain, leaving his audience to guess what this meant—and to assume the worst.

Next came a cooking demonstration—essentially a video version of the EWG report—in which Houlihan fried bacon to show that Teflon releases toxic fumes at normal temperatures. Never mind that there was no analysis of the air during this demonstration, nor did Ross bother to question whether this method of cooking bacon was a fair representation of reality. He simply informed viewers that "the hotter it gets, the more chemicals are released."

Further echoing EWG's report, Ross insinuated that there was some kind of cover-up involving Teflon flu. "It turns out," he said in a "gotcha" tone, "this Teflon flu is something DuPont has known about for years." Had he included any medical experts as sources, he might have learned that doctors are well aware of this "secret," which has been documented in the medical literature.

Instead, he left it to Chowdhry to explain the condition, again challenging her assertions with a smart-aleck attitude:

Chowdhry: "You feel like you have the flu temporarily."
Ross: "And how long does that last?"
Chowdhry: "Temporary. Couple days."
Ross: "Couple days?"
Chowdhry: "A couple days."
Ross: "That's temporarily?"

From there, the reporter moved on to the threat to birds. Sounding like a lawyer for EWG conducting a cross-examination, he asked Chowdhry: "In West Virginia, they used to use birds in coal mines as a warning of problems. Is this not the same thing?"

Not satisfied with her answer, he followed up: "But if it will kill a bird, wouldn't it at the very least do some harm to a tiny baby?"

When Chowdhry responded, "There is no evidence that it causes harm," he shot back, "But as a scientist, doesn't that seem logical to you?"

The time devoted to this unenlightening exchange would have been much better spent hearing from an independent veterinarian or physician who had studied the issue. But they would have likely thrown cold water on EWG's "canary in a coal mine" reasoning, getting in the way of Ross's storyline and his chance to go after a corporate bad guy.

The final part of the segment returned to Bucky Bailey's story and that of another woman who attributed her child's birth defect to the DuPont plant. Portraying these anecdotes as evidence, Ross closed by tying Bailey's experience to the question of "whether the Teflon chemical that's in everyone's blood is safe."

Following EWG's lead, Ross had taken three separate issues—the ubiquity of PFOA, Teflon flu, and allegations regarding the plant—and misleadingly linked them in an attempt to incriminate Teflon and DuPont. Had Ross thoroughly and truthfully covered the story, he would have made these points clear:

- PFOA is ubiquitous in the environment, and there's concern (though no direct evidence) that it may cause harm to humans. Scientists are still not sure whether the levels in most of our bodies are high enough to pose a threat. Though they don't fully understand how we're exposed to PFOA, it's likely that very little, if any, of our exposure comes from Teflon pots and pans.

- Cooking with Teflon has long been recognized to harm birds and, in rare cases, to cause flulike symptoms in people. Everyone should be aware of these possibilities and take precautions such as using proper ventilation and avoiding very high cooking temperatures.

- DuPont failed to tell the government everything it knew about elevated PFOA levels in drinking water near the Teflon plant and in the blood of workers and nearby residents. It's quite possible that they have suffered harm, as they allege. But because epidemiological studies to date have not found an association, no one can say for certain. This concern, however, has little or nothing to do with risks to consumers (or their birds) posed by Teflon-coated cookware.

By failing to include independent experts to explain these subtleties and provide perspective, the segment served as propaganda for EWG, making its case more forcefully than the group could itself. It's no surprise that an ABC News promotional press release, headlined "Brian Ross Reports on Concerns that a Key Chemical Used in the Manufacture of Teflon Might Pose Health Risks," was proudly posted on EWG's Web site. By reducing this highly complicated matter to a simplistic villain-victim-vindicator narrative, the segment made for compelling television and was a boon to EWG's cause—but not to our understanding of the issue.

Two years later, Ross was back on the air with another EWG-inspired exposé on Teflon, this one involving food packaging. Viewers of *Good Morning America* awoke to the unappetizing news that a chemical called Zonyl RP, which is in the lining of food containers such as candy wrappers, pizza boxes, and microwave popcorn bags, might pose a health hazard by leaching into food and breaking down into PFOA in our bodies.

The report came after an EWG press conference and news release announcing that, according to a former DuPont chemical engineer, the company "hid for decades that it was polluting Americans' blood with a hyper-persistent chemical associated with grease-resistant coatings on paper food packaging." Ross's report prominently featured the whistleblower, Glen Evers, who alleged that "you don't see it, you don't feel it, you can't taste it, but when you open that bag and you start dipping your French fries in there . . . you are eating it." Evers went on to explain that this is "a very bad thing" because "the chemical goes into the blood, and it stays there for a very long period of time."

Ross cited a DuPont memo obtained by EWG, which supposedly revealed that "the chemical was coming off at three times what the FDA allowed." That was followed by a sound bite from an EWG official who— to no one's surprise—denounced DuPont, accusing it of "a pattern of cover-up and suppression." Consistent with his previous reporting, Ross didn't challenge the assertions by EWG or Evers, nor did he bother to include interviews with independent scientists or the FDA.

Had he done more homework, Ross would have learned that EWG's allegations were baseless. A month after the report, the FDA informed EWG in a letter that the supposedly incriminating memo it had uncovered was "irrelevant to the safety determination on the use of Zonyl RP." It turned out that, according to DuPont's most rigorous tests, levels of exposure to the chemical were actually 45 times *lower* than the safety threshold cited by EWG. Like the confused tirades by Gilda Radner's old *Saturday Night Live* character Emily Litella, the factually challenged allegations by EWG and Ross ended with a "never mind"—only Ross never acknowledged this to his viewers.

A few months later, Ross had yet another story on Teflon—this time regarding the EPA's announcement that, given the potential but unproven threat from PFOA, it was asking companies to eliminate PFOA emissions, just to be safe. The *World News Tonight* piece, which portrayed the chemical as a proven hazard, featured Bucky Bailey's mother, Sue, who called the development a "bittersweet victory."

This angle mirrored EWG's press release, which commended the Baileys for having "the courage to stand up in public to raise health concerns about these chemicals" (they and other residents near the DuPont plant had sued the company) and referred to the "bittersweet promise" that the EPA's action would reduce future health damage from PFOA.

On *World News Tonight*, Ross did not mention the lack of hard evidence for the Baileys' assertions. Nor did he include the EPA administrator's statement, issued at a press conference, that "to date EPA is not aware of any studies specifically relating current levels of PFOA exposure to human health effects." Instead, at the end of the story, Ross told viewers that, according to the government, there's no need "right now" to throw out Teflon pots and pans. Elizabeth Vargas, the program's anchor, responded, "No need to throw them out, but it seems like plenty of need for concern." Anyone not familiar with the science who had seen Ross's unbalanced presentation would have agreed with Vargas.

To be sure, Ross wasn't the only journalist who fell under EWG's sway and mangled the Teflon story. But he seemed to do so with greater gusto than just about anyone else, devoting more attention to it and making it one of his pet issues. Indeed, when he reported the EPA announcement on *Good Morning America*, the program's co-host noted, "Brian, you've been on this story from the very beginning." Unfortunately for viewers, his tenacity never led him to the truth.

Trevor Butterworth of the Statistical Assessment Service (STATS), a group affiliated with George Mason University that identifies and comments on scientific misinformation in the media, has written extensively about the coverage of Teflon and PFOA. He observes that these and other activist-generated stories about chemicals are generally not "reported in a way that tries to evaluate their truth by looking at the science." Instead, journalists often assume that by including "the other side" from industry spokespersons—whose comments invariably come across as predictable and self-serving—they've done their jobs. "The question," asks Butterworth, is "whether journalists are doing the public any favors by giving these watchdogs a soapbox instead of doing some fact checking and seeking out independent expert testimony."

So why do journalists report these stories in such a way? For one thing, they frequently don't know where to turn for expert guidance, much less how to dissect the science. Also, many reporters see themselves as natural allies of activists, as they're both in the business of uncovering wrongdoing and enlightening the public. Then there's journalists' irresistible attraction to stories about things that threaten us. In his book *Myths, Lies, and Downright Stupidity*, ABC's John Stossel—the co-host of *20/20*, which aired one of Brian Ross's scare stories on Teflon—explains that reporters "know that the scarier and more bizarre the story, the more likely it is that our bosses will give us more air time or a front-page slot. The scary story, justified or not, will get higher ratings and sell more papers. Fear sells."

FOUL-SMELLING CLAIMS

One consequence of this fear-mongering over risks that are merely theoretical—and, if they exist, likely quite small—is that it can skew our priorities. Take, for example, warnings about new car smell. A Michigan-based activist group known as the Ecology Center alleges that toxic fumes are being emitted from chemicals used to make steering wheels, seats, and dashboards. The group claims that when drivers and passengers inhale or ingest these substances, the results can be serious health problems, including allergic reactions, birth defects, liver toxicity, and cancer.

It's true that some chemicals used to make car interiors are known to give off volatile organic compounds (VOCs), which have been linked to adverse health effects, including what's sometimes called "sick building syndrome." Some research has found relatively high VOC levels in new, parked cars that are hot from the sun, but these levels rapidly decline when the autos are cooled off and ventilated.

As for direct evidence that car interiors cause harm, none exists. In one study, a team of German researchers heated two parked cars—one new and another three years old—to 150 degrees F. After collecting air samples and exposing them to human and animal cells, they concluded that the new car might slightly aggravate certain allergies. Otherwise, they found "no apparent health hazard of parked motor vehicle indoor air."

This kind of careful research, in which chemical exposure levels and their effects are measured, is necessary to determine the true extent of any health problems from car interiors. But that's not the approach of the Ecology Center. Instead, it has created and publicized the "Consumer Guide to Toxic Chemicals in Cars," which ranks autos according to the chemical health hazards they allegedly pose. The group compiled its report by analyzing the chemical makeup of 15 components from cars, including steering wheels, dashboards, seats, and carpeting. It didn't bother, however, to determine whether drivers and passengers are actually exposed to these chemicals, how high the exposure levels are, and whether they're harmful. Instead, it assumed that the mere presence of chemicals leads to harm—a breathtaking leap of scientific logic.

The group's exaggeration of the certainty and size of this risk can distort our perspective about dangers posed by cars. When it comes to air inside autos, a real and well-documented threat to our health is from exhaust fumes emitted by other vehicles. Numerous studies suggest that cars may contain hazardous levels of benzene, carbon monoxide, and other substances, especially during rush hour on congested roads.

Even that threat pales in comparison to the risk of injury and death due to car accidents. More than 2.5 million Americans are injured every year as a result of vehicle crashes, and about 43,000 are killed—a death toll roughly equal to that from falls, HIV/AIDS, and gun assaults *combined*. Vehicle accidents are the leading single cause of death in people under 35. Now those are statistics truly worth worrying about.

When activist groups alarm us over far lesser—and perhaps nonexistent—threats, we can quickly lose sight of the big picture. We may end up

obsessing over what chemicals are wafting from our car seats, while thinking nothing of speeding or distracting ourselves by talking on cell phones
while driving. Similarly, we may panic over the possibility that our fast-food
containers are leaching dangerous chemicals, heedless of the fact that the
double burgers, triple-cheese pizzas, and supersized fries in those containers are what really threaten our health.

BARKING DOGS

One reason for this irrationality is that we're more likely to fear something
if it's unfamiliar or outside our control. Unlike risks we know about and
often willingly accept, such as driving a car or eating an unhealthful diet,
exposing ourselves to chemicals in cosmetics, cookware, or cars isn't something we generally choose to do. It's foisted upon us without our consent or
even our knowledge. Activists are well aware of this and exploit our tendency to overreact to such threats.

As hard as it might be, we need to avoid succumbing to this urge and to
keep activists' alerts about chemicals in perspective. That entails remembering a few key principles:

- ANIMALS AREN'T PEOPLE. While studies of lab animals can be useful for
  identifying potentially harmful chemicals, they don't necessarily apply
  to people. Extrapolating findings from animal studies to predict risk in
  humans can be highly misleading.
- DOSE MATTERS. Even the most benign substance can be toxic if enough
  of it is ingested. Simply because something poses a health risk at a high
  dose doesn't necessarily mean it's harmful in small amounts.
- NOT ALL RISKS ARE CREATED EQUAL. When we hear, for example, that a substance may "increase the risk of cancer," we should ask, "By how
  much?" A chemical associated with a tiny rise in the absolute risk of a
  rare cancer, for instance, is less cause for concern than something
  linked to a substantial increase in the risk of a more common cancer.

As much as we may admire and appreciate activists' crusading spirit—
and they certainly deserve credit for bringing certain health and envi-

ronmental issues to light—we shouldn't give them a pass. When they make exaggerated claims and we take these at face value, we may not only become unnecessarily frightened but also end up with misplaced health priorities. It's nice to have watchdogs looking out for us, but it's up to us to decide whether they're barking at the right things.

TRUSTWORTHY SOURCES OF INFORMATION

Statistical Assessment Service, STATS (www.stats.org). This organization analyzes the use of statistics and science in the media regarding a variety of issues, including chemicals and health. Though criticized by some for its ties to the Center for Media and Public Affairs, a conservative-leaning media research organization, STATS provides independent, nonideological critiques of news reports, setting the record straight. The Web site includes links to other useful resources.

ToxNet (www.nlm.nih.gov/pubs/factsheets/toxnetfs.html). Managed by the National Library of Medicine, this is a cluster of databases, all of which offer information on potentially hazardous chemicals and the risks they pose to humans.

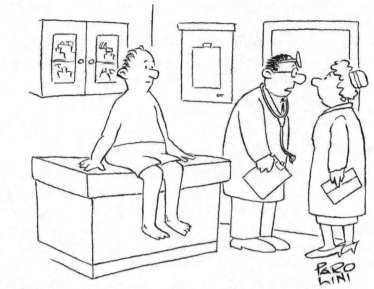

www.CartoonStock.com

" HIS BIOLOGICAL CLOCK NEEDS REWINDING."

CHAPTER NINE: ANTI-AGING DOCTORS
DON'T GET SICK, DON'T GET OLD, DON'T DIE!

They bill themselves as "the #1 preventative, anti-aging medical society in the world." So when I learned that the American Academy of Anti-Aging Medicine, or A4M, would be holding another of their regular conferences, I naturally was interested in attending and called to let them know. Their response caught me by surprise: You're not invited.

In my twenty years as a health journalist, I have sat in on countless scientific meetings, and all have welcomed me with open arms. Many even set aside working areas for reporters and offer press releases and tip sheets to highlight studies that might be of special interest. A4M, in contrast, was turning journalists (or at least this one) away. When I asked why, I was told, "We don't owe you an explanation." Hmm. Perhaps they had figured out that I wrote a regular newspaper column dissecting dubious health claims. Did they have something to hide? Determined to find out, I signed up as a nonjournalist (the general public was welcome, even though certain journalists weren't) and paid the registration fee.

At the meeting, I found several thousand people, most of them physicians and other providers who practice "anti-aging" medicine or would like to. In a giant auditorium, they listened with rapt attention as A4M's cofounder and chairman, Dr. Robert Goldman, reviewed the three "rules" of this field: 1. Don't get sick. 2. Don't get old. 3. Don't die. Goldman, whose claim to fame includes world records for consecutive sit-ups, handstand push-ups, and other athletic feats, predicted that many in the audience would live to be 100 and that, thanks to medical advances, life expectancies well beyond 100—even as high as 150—were soon to come.

A parade of other speakers addressed topics ranging from heavy metal detoxification to hair replacement. While some presented interesting data from seemingly sound studies, others expounded on their own unproven and sometimes bizarre theories. Overall, the most frequently discussed subject was the use of hormones such as testosterone, DHEA, and human growth hormone for countering aging.

Attendees learned how, while increasing their patients' life spans, they could also increase their own profits—a goal that clearly had attracted many to this meeting. Indeed, in a promotional brochure for an upcoming conference, A4M listed "Learn hands on income generating . . . procedures" and "Expand your cash practice" as two of the top five reasons to attend.

The meeting I attended included an exhibit hall filled with vendors hawking a huge array of products and services, some legitimate and many others that were questionable at best. Among my favorites: a foot bath device that allegedly could detoxify the entire body, and a laser that was touted as a way to help you "lose weight NOW!!" A number of booths promoted dietary supplements that could supposedly increase energy, boost brain power, improve libido, reduce stress, or grow hair. One company selling such supplements held out the promise of $50,000 or more in annual income for doctors who referred patients.

With the disclaimer that the products "have not been evaluated or approved by A4M," the group encouraged attendees to "exercise your personal scrutiny, educated and demanding scientific evaluation in assessing the ideas and products presented." But given the unalloyed enthusiasm displayed by many attendees for ideas that should have raised eyebrows, there didn't seem to be much "scrutiny" or "demanding scientific evaluation" going on in either the exhibit hall or the sessions. Unlike most other scientific conferences, where theories and opinions are vigorously challenged and debated, this was a gathering for true believers. As my persona non grata status suggested, it was not a place where healthy skeptics were especially welcome.

What I encountered at this meeting—sound ideas mixed with unproven ones and a tendency to embrace them all with equal fervor—is typical of what you often get from anti-aging doctors and clinics. While some of their advice—eat a proper diet, exercise, don't smoke—is backed up by solid science, much of what they push is not. It can be hard to resist promises of eternal youth from people in white coats who claim to be at the leading edge of preventive medicine. But as healthy skeptics, we need to make sure the edge they're luring us onto isn't in fact a limb with inadequate support.

IFFY ASSERTIONS

The term "anti-aging" can have different meanings depending on who's using it. For example, some self-described anti-aging clinics are devoted mainly or exclusively to cosmetic surgery. The ones to which I refer, however, focus on longevity and wellness, offering what one clinic calls "internal plastic surgery." Sometimes these doctors and clinics use terms such as "age management," "life extension," or simply "prevention" instead of "anti-aging." Whatever the case, their promises tend to be similar:

"Reverse the effects of aging"

"Turn back the hands of time"

"Reset your biological clock"

"Slow the rate at which you age"

"Restore and maintain youthful vigor"

"Prolong your life and health span, as well as your quality of life"

The process typically begins with extensive blood work to measure levels of various hormones, nutrients, and other substances. Patients may also be given a battery of tests for things such as bone density, lean body mass, skin elasticity, metabolic rate, and mental function. Clinics often refer to such measurements as "biomarkers" of aging, which supposedly indicate your "real" age, as opposed to your chronological one. The problem is that there's no scientific consensus on what constitutes a valid biomarker of aging. A panel of gerontology experts convened to study the issue concluded that any claims to measure such biomarkers "are not scientifically based." Dr. Robert Butler, the panel's leader and one of the nation's most respected authorities on aging, has summed it up this way: "We simply do not have the equivalent of a blood pressure cuff for testing aging."

Nevertheless, clinics use such measurements as the basis for what they call "precise and customized" anti-aging treatments, which often include dietary supplements, especially antioxidants. The theory is that free radicals can harm cells and cause aging, and that antioxidants such as vitamins A, C, and E neutralize free radicals. Animal and observational studies have suggested that higher intakes of antioxidants through diet may help protect against heart disease and cancer. And solid research has shown that antioxidant supplements may help slow the development of macular degeneration, a leading cause of blindness in older people.

But most clinical trials putting antioxidant supplements to the test have found no benefits. A review of the evidence by a team of British scientists concluded that, in general, the use of supplements as anti-aging treatments "is not supported by the currently available scientific literature." And a study published in the *Journal of the American Medical Association*, which pooled results from a number of trials, concluded that taking vitamin A and E supplements was associated with a slightly *increased* risk of dying earlier. As discussed in chapter 4, the same was true for the antioxidant beta-carotene.

Despite these research findings, anti-aging clinics frequently instruct patients to take as many as several dozen antioxidant and other supplement pills a day. Some practitioners sell supplements in their offices or on their Web sites. The ubiquitous presence of vitamin and herb hucksters at A4M meetings further attests to the central role of supplements in anti-aging medicine, as does the A4M Web site, which links visitors to a supplement-selling service peddling "physician-picked" products ranging from oregano oil to green tea extract.

Robert Goldman and A4M's other founder, Dr. Ronald Klatz, have even developed their own anti-aging supplements, an accomplishment that earned them a mock award from three scientists, including S. Jay Olshansky, a University of Illinois professor of epidemiology who's an expert on the demographics of aging. Known as the "silver fleece" award, it's a bottle labeled "snake oil" given to the product with the "most ridiculous, outrageous, scientifically unsupported or exaggerated assertions" about fighting aging. Pointing out that "there are no known dietary supplements that have been proven to alter the aging process," Olshansky adds, "About the only thing these anti-aging products do is fatten the wallets of those selling them."

HORMONES AS HEALTH ENHANCERS

Another pillar of anti-aging medicine—and its most controversial feature—is the liberal use of certain hormones. As we age, levels of these hormones decline, a process associated with decreased strength, muscle mass, skin thickness, bone density, and sex drive as well as increased body fat. It's been shown that replenishing hormones, at least in the short term, can positively affect some of these changes. But a number of questions remain: How large are these improvements? How long do they last? Are they strictly cosmetic, or do they result in physiologically younger bodies that are less susceptible to age-related diseases? What are the risks and side effects?

You typically don't hear about these uncertainties from anti-aging clinics. Instead, they trumpet benefits that often sound miraculous, especially in reference to human growth hormone (GH), a genetically engineered prescription drug that's administered by injection. For example, one popular clinic lists the following effects of GH:

"Rejuvinates [sic] every cell in the body"

"Helps the body heal faster"

"Strengthens bones"

"Boosts energy to youthful levels"

What's more, GH replacement will supposedly give you "restorative sleep," "skin rejuvenation and rapid wound healing," "improved memory, alertness, and concentration span," "improved immunity," "vital organ re-growth," and a "sense of well-being."

As evidence for these seemingly magical effects, anti-aging doctors and clinics often cite a 1990 *New England Journal of Medicine* study (mentioned in chapter 4), in which GH was administered to twelve healthy older men for six months. The subjects experienced an increase in lean body mass and skin thickness and a decrease in body fat. Adverse effects included small increases in blood pressure and glucose levels. Because the study was small and preliminary, the lead author, Dr. Daniel Rudman of the Medical College of Wisconsin, pointed out that more questions needed to be answered "before the possible benefits of human growth hormone in the elderly can be explored." An accompanying editorial expressed similar caution, concluding that "because there are so many unanswered questions about the use of growth hormone in the elderly . . . its general use now or in the immediate future is not justified."

The caveats seemed to fall on deaf ears among anti-aging enthusiasts, who seized on the study as the scientific basis for their new movement. In the dedication of his 1997 book, *Grow Young with HGH*, A4M's Ronald Klatz went so far as to credit the work of Dr. Rudman, who died in 1994, for marking "the beginning of the end of aging, and the birth of the 'ageless society.'"

Subsequent research has reinforced the need for caution, with studies finding decreases in body fat among those taking GH, but no statistically significant improvements in strength, endurance, or mental function. Side effects included swelling, joint pain, carpal tunnel syndrome, glucose intolerance, and diabetes.

Some scientists fear that an additional adverse effect might be the growth of cancer. That's because growth hormone stimulates production of a substance called insulinlike growth factor, or IGF-1, and elevated levels of IGF-1 have been associated with an increased risk of breast, prostate, and colon cancer. While no studies to date have found a direct link between GH and cancer in humans, this theoretical risk should be regarded as at least a possibility until long-term studies demonstrate otherwise.

Anti-aging doctors dismiss the link to cancer and claim that they don't see any of the side effects found in research studies because they use lower doses and space them out over a longer period. But since these regimens haven't been subjected to rigorous long-term trials, it's impossible to know whether they're safe and effective. Most of the studies cited by anti-aging doctors to prove their case have limited relevance because they don't involve healthy older people with age-related declines in levels—the types of patients who typically visit anti-aging clinics.

In addition to its use for increasing height in short children, GH medication is FDA-approved for treating adults with growth hormone deficiency, a relatively rare condition involving an abnormality of the pituitary gland, where GH is produced. The condition is diagnosed by endocrinologists according to strict criteria. Because it's illegal to distribute GH for nonapproved purposes—which include anti-aging treatments—many anti-aging doctors are careful to claim that they prescribe it to treat growth hormone deficiency. But their standards for determining who qualifies as GH deficient tend to be far less stringent than those used by endocrinologists, and many of their patients who would normally be considered healthy end up with the diagnosis.

Indeed, the controversial notion that naturally declining GH levels constitute a "disease" warranting treatment lies at the core of anti-aging medicine. Mainstream scientists raise the possibility that just the opposite is true: the age-related drop in GH may be protective. Mice with deficiencies of growth hormone actually live *longer* than those with higher levels, and it could be that our decreasing GH as we age is nature's way of helping us fend off disease and death. This, too, is just a theory, however. Research is under way to get more definitive answers, and until they're in, no one knows for certain whether boosting GH levels in healthy older people is, in the long run, helpful or harmful. Anyone who uses the drug as an anti-aging tonic is therefore taking a gamble.

The same is true for testosterone, another favorite hormone of anti-aging practitioners, which is prescribed to both men and women. In men, levels decline gradually and steadily with age. Anti-aging doctors assert that replacing testosterone to youthful levels can produce dramatic effects; one clinic claims, for example, that "libido and improved mood return within days" and that "regrowth of muscle and bone occurs within months."

In fact, some randomized studies do suggest that testosterone replacement may positively affect body fat, bone density, muscle strength, sexual functioning, and general well-being in older men who are mildly deficient. But most studies are small and short-term, and not all show such improvements. As for risks, research shows that testosterone replacement can stimulate benign growth of the prostate gland and increase PSA, a possible marker for prostate cancer (discussed in chapter 6). Though there's no direct evidence that testosterone promotes prostate cancer, some scientists believe it's a possibility, based on what's known about the effects of testosterone. Likewise, others express theoretical concerns that testosterone may increase the risk of heart disease, though some research suggests that it may reduce cholesterol levels and lead to certain improvements in people with heart problems. An analysis that pooled data from 30 trials found no evidence of cardiovascular effects (either harmful or beneficial), but the lack of long-term research means the truth, at this point, is anyone's guess.

An expert panel convened by the Institute of Medicine concluded that there are too many unknowns to justify using testosterone therapy to combat aging and that more research is needed. "Until the efficacy and safety of testosterone therapy in older men is firmly established," said the panel's leader, "we believe that its use is appropriate only for those conditions approved by the FDA." These include hypogonadism, an extreme deficiency in testosterone production that is different from the normal decline associated with aging.

Many anti-aging doctors also put great faith in dehydroepiandrosterone (DHEA), a hormone that's converted in the body to testosterone and estrogen. Levels in both men and women begin to fall after age 30; by age 60, levels are half what they were in young adulthood. Some observational studies have found an association between higher levels of DHEA and lower rates of cardiovascular death in men, but not in women.

Small, short-term studies in healthy older people, measuring outcomes such as mood, insulin sensitivity, body composition, and bone density, have produced mixed results. In a two-year randomized study published in the *New England Journal of Medicine*, men and women who received DHEA had a small decrease in body fat and an increase in bone density. But they had no improvements in physical performance (as measured by muscle strength and aerobic capacity), insulin sensitivity, or quality of life.

The fact that the FDA classifies DHEA as a dietary supplement, not a drug, has prompted one anti-aging clinic to declare that "DHEA is so safe and relatively free of side effects that the FDA does not require a prescription for its sale." That's highly misleading. While it's true that studies—including the one in the *New England Journal of Medicine*—have so far found no major side effects from DHEA, that's not why it's considered a dietary supplement. The FDA banned DHEA in 1985, but the action was overturned by the controversial 1994 Dietary Supplement Health and Education Act (described in chapter 4), which stripped the FDA of its power to strictly regulate the substance.

Some scientists see that change as a big mistake, especially given their concern that DHEA might stimulate the growth of cancer. As with testosterone and GH, such a risk is only theoretical. But as one review of the scientific evidence concluded, "This issue needs to be fully addressed in long-term studies in humans."

Rounding out the anti-aging armamentarium are the hormones estrogen and progesterone. Their inclusion may come as a surprise, given that the large Women's Health Initiative clinical trial found that the risks of long-term hormone replacement therapy—breast cancer, heart attacks, strokes, and blood clots—may outweigh the benefits for many women. But anti-aging doctors often insist that the hormones they prescribe are different, a "much better form of HRT," as one clinic puts it.

Conventional forms of HRT, which were used in the Women's Health Initiative, include synthetic progesterone (known as progestin) as well as mixtures of horse and human estrogens. By contrast, the versions prescribed by many anti-aging doctors, so-called natural or bioidentical hormones, are made from plants and more closely resemble hormones in the human body. They may come in the form of pills, patches, or creams. Though these products in some cases are manufactured and dispensed like any other drug, they may also be prepared by special compounding pharmacies that can custom-mix ingredients for each patient. Anti-aging doctors often use compounding pharmacies as their source for estrogen and progesterone, as well as for DHEA and "natural" testosterone.

Many consumers have heard of bioidentical hormones, thanks to actress Suzanne Somers, whose best-selling books tout their purported benefits.

Siding with Somers (the same person, as I mentioned in chapter 3, who promotes scientifically baseless diet advice) and sometimes even invoking her on their Web sites, anti-aging doctors claim that these hormones don't pose the same risks as conventional HRT. The reason, according to one clinic, is that "the body accepts and metabolizes natural hormones as if it made them." This clinic echoes many others in its claim that bioidentical hormones have been "proven" to help women "lose weight, reinvigorate their sex lives, build bone density, improve mood, and fight the symptoms of aging."

In reality, little long-term research on bioidentical hormones has been conducted, and no definitive evidence exists that they're safer or more effective than conventional HRT. What's more, because preparations from compounding pharmacies aren't regulated by the FDA as standard prescription drugs are, there's no way to be sure about their purity and potency. An FDA analysis of 29 product samples from compounding pharmacies found that 10 of them—about one-third—failed at least one quality test. This compares with an overall failure rate of less than 2 percent for standard drugs.

It's ironic that many anti-aging practitioners point to the Women's Health Initiative study to support their case that bioidentical hormones are superior to conventional HRT. In fact, what the WHI teaches us is not to jump to conclusions without sufficient evidence—the very thing these doctors and clinics are guilty of doing. If nothing else, the lesson from decades of research is that giving hormones to healthy people is fraught with complexity. There may indeed be benefits, but those have to be weighed against side effects and risks that can be serious and even life-threatening. Only through long-term clinical trials can we have anything close to a full understanding of what all these risks and benefits actually are and how they stack up against each other.

It may well turn out that the hormones embraced by anti-aging doctors—whether estrogen, progesterone, testosterone, DHEA, or growth hormone—have benefits that outweigh the risks. But then again, maybe not. Right now, we have no way to be sure. When anti-aging doctors and clinics suggest otherwise—with statements, for example, that hormone therapy is "safe and has no adverse effects" and that "the positive benefits of it are overwhelming"—they foolishly repeat the mistakes of those who jumped the gun regarding conventional HRT. Patients who listen to them may end up unwittingly taking chances that they wouldn't if they had all the facts.

CALL TODAY FOR AN APPOINTMENT!

The desire to avoid aging and restore lost youth is, by itself, enough to attract many consumers to anti-aging clinics. But adding to the allure are certain highly touted features of these practices.

EXTRA ATTENTION

Typically, doctors at these clinics give you far more time and attention than you get with conventional medical care. Initial consultations in some practices last for two hours, followed by the opportunity for multiple follow-up visits and continuous access to doctors through phone calls and e-mails. Many clinics use the word "comprehensive" to emphasize their focus on your overall health and well-being—something that's too often lacking in conventional medicine.

But there's a steep cost for this extra care. An initial evaluation and lab tests can run well over $1,000. Then you often have a yearly "professional" or "maintenance" fee, which can be up to several thousand dollars or more, depending on how much ongoing attention you want and need. On top of that, there's the cost for treatment. One clinic, for example, charges more than $300 for a year's supply of DHEA, $900 for testosterone, and $1,200 for supplements. The price for growth hormone can be as high as $12,000 a year.

For a comprehensive treatment program that includes all or most of what a clinic offers, you can easily shell out $15,000 or more a year. And because the effects from hormones tend to go away if you stop taking them, you need to stay on the program—and keep paying—indefinitely. Insurance typically does not cover the vast majority of the costs.

BOARD-CERTIFIED DOCTORS

To enhance their credibility, many anti-aging clinics emphasize that their doctors are board-certified in anti-aging medicine. The certification program, which is offered by A4M, involves a written and oral exam. Those who pay a fee and pass the written test earn the designation of "diplomate" in anti-aging medicine. Practitioners who go on to pass the oral exam as well may refer to themselves as "board-certified." Though anti-aging doctors would like you to believe otherwise, this credential doesn't carry the same weight as board certification in mainstream disciplines such as internal medicine, ophthalmology, or orthopedic surgery. The A4M credential is not recognized by the American Board of Medical Specialties, which sets standards for certification for more than 130 specialties and subspecialties.

Unlike other fields, which require several (if not many) years of residency training for board certification, anti-aging medicine has no such prerequisite. Instead, doctors need continuing medical education credits in an area such as preventive medicine or nutrition (which can be earned by attending lectures or taking online courses), along with five years of clinical experience in any field of medicine. The materials that candidates must master for exams consist largely of books written by A4M's founders, Ronald Klatz and Robert Goldman, both of whom earned their MDs from the Central America Health Sciences University in Belize. Neither has residency training in geriatrics or endocrinology.

Alternatively, some doctors advertise that they are "certified in clinical age management." Offered by a chain of clinics known as Cenegenics, this program involves studying materials at home, attending a one-week training session, and taking a multiple-choice exam, which virtually everyone passes. Those who successfully meet these requirements receive a certificate indicating that they have the "training and qualifications" to practice age management medicine.

Though Cenegenics shuns the term "anti-aging" and is not affiliated with A4M, both organizations describe the benefits of their certification programs in similar ways. Cenegenics urges doctors to become certified in order to "break free from the medical insurance maze" and "boost your income." Likewise, A4M calls board certification "your gateway to opportunity" and lists "increase your practice's annual income" as a top reason for getting certified. Such rhetoric is worth keeping in mind whenever you see anti-aging doctors touting their credentials.

SATISFIED PATIENTS

In some cases, clinics promote the success of their therapies with testimonials from satisfied customers. For example, a publication from Cenegenics is filled with quotes from patients such as these:

> "My body fat is now 12%, down from 32% a year ago. My strength and muscle mass are at the highest level I've ever had in my life! My bone density (hips/spine) has improved to normal. My skin looks at least ten years younger. My libido and sexual energy are like when I was in my 30s."

> "I wish I had a picture of me last year, but I refused to have any taken. I was so bedraggled, fat, bloated and stressed. Now I'm clear, together, calm, and finding pleasure in everything."

> "Thanks to Cenegenics, I'm feeling and looking great . . . while aging younger!"

Likewise, newspaper ads for Cenegenics feature a photo of an older shirtless man—who is Cenegenics's head doctor—with a bodybuilder physique. In large, bold letters, one ad asks, "Why does this 67-year-old man have the body of a 30-year-old?" Another, which has run frequently in the *New York Times*, inquires, "How does this doctor look better than ever and stay healthy year after year?" The answer: Cenegenics's "unique and balanced combination" of diet, exercise, and hormones. "This doctor's results speak for themselves," we're told.

One problem with these and other testimonials is their tendency to confuse appearance and health. Good looks and good health are not necessarily the same. As research on hormones has shown, you can gain muscle and lose fat without increasing your strength or stamina. Put another way, you can develop a chiseled physique and remain relatively unhealthy. Likewise, you can be in excellent health without having flat abs, thin thighs, or bulging biceps. Testimonials touting lean, muscular bodies therefore do not "speak for themselves" when it comes to healthy aging.

Another dilemma is knowing what's responsible for the person's improved health and well-being. When hormones, supplements, diet, and exercise are used simultaneously, as is often the case at clinics, it can be difficult, if not impossible, to sort out the effects of each. Patients featured in testimonials may attribute their newfound energy and vigor to hormones and supplements. But it could be that (cost-free) changes in diet and exercise, which are also part of their regimens, actually deserve the credit. Of course, those who have spent thousands of dollars on anti-aging programs are unlikely to believe this. And beliefs—not evidence—are what testimonials are all about.

SCIENTISTS SPEAK OUT

In an effort to set the record straight, Jay Olshansky, the University of Illinois professor cited earlier in this chapter, teamed up with Leonard Hayflick, an acclaimed gerontology researcher at the University of California, San Francisco, and Bruce Carnes, an assistant professor of geriatric medicine at the University of Oklahoma, to craft a science-based statement about human aging. Published on the *Scientific American* Web site in 2002, it was endorsed by 48 other scientists, including leading researchers in the field of aging. The statement minced no words about anti-aging remedies: "The more dramatic claims made by those who advocate antiaging medicine in the form of specific drugs, vitamin cocktails or esoteric hormone mixtures . . . are not supported by scientific evidence, and it is difficult to avoid the conclusion that these claims are intentionally false, misleading or exaggerated for commercial reasons."

Pointing out that "since recorded history individuals have been, and are continuing to be, victimized by promises of extended youth or increased longevity," the authors urged the public to "avoid buying or using products or other interventions from anyone claiming that they will slow, stop or reverse aging."

It was a message that some didn't want to hear. Many consumers who read about it in an AARP publication posted negative—even angry—

responses on the organization's Internet message boards. "I will not heed their warnings," said one defiant poster, while another wrote: "There are MOUNTAINS of evidence that show many of the therapies and products derided in this article help people like me live more active lives." Opined yet another: "There are more scientists alive and working than ever lived on this planet before. Just because you got 51 of them to make some claim does not make it significant."

These responses reflect the unshakable faith that some people put in measures like supplements and hormones, no matter how inconclusive the evidence. Challenging their beliefs elicits the kind of indignant reaction you might get from questioning someone else's religion.

This resistance also stems from the deeply rooted desire, born of our fear of aging and death, to escape the infirmities and indignities of old age. For many, the possibility that we can control how we age and experience our later years is a source of great comfort. Anyone who shatters that hope by telling us there's nothing we can do—which was not the scientists' message but was nevertheless how many readers perceived it—is likely to be met with jeers.

Predictably, A4M's response to the scientific statement was even more ferocious. After all, it wasn't just their members' beliefs that were under attack but also their very livelihoods. Issuing a document that read more like a screed than a scientific defense, A4M lashed out at the scientists' statement as a "propaganda campaign" by the "gerontological establishment," which they labeled a "death cult of gerontology" that "seeks to silence the most visible independent source of innovation in aging research and education."

Indeed, the notion that they are persecuted pioneers battling the forces of darkness is a favorite theme of anti-aging doctors. Often they liken themselves to Galileo (no one can accuse them of excess modesty) and other heroes of science who were vilified by their contemporaries but later vindicated. When you hear this, keep in mind that for every maverick like Galileo who turned out to be right, there were far more whose ideas were proven wrong—especially when it comes to aging. As for A4M's conspiracy theories, the truth is that the "gerontological establishment," which is far from monolithic, is aggressively pursuing all kinds of research leads involving potential life-extenders, ranging from calorie restriction to substances in red wine. Unlike anti-aging practitioners, however, these scientists are subjecting their ideas to rigorous study before drawing definitive conclusions. Ironically, anti-aging medicine stands to benefit greatly if this work by the "establishment" it denounces ends up panning out.

In A4M's response to the *Scientific American* statement, you can also find another pet idea of anti-aging medicine: that the dramatic rise in life expectancy during the last century is evidence that we're headed toward "practical immortality." In its statement, the group quotes the chairman of a business-consulting group who observes: "Looking at historical trends, one finds that over the past century, we nearly doubled our lifespan . . . There's no reason to imagine that we won't do at least as much in the next century. If you double 85, you're at 170 . . ."

This is a demographic leap of logic. In 1900, the average life expectancy in the United States was about 47. Today it's nearly 80. As impressive as this is—it's the largest and most rapid longevity gain in recorded human history—the statistics can be misleading. It's not as though most people who lived a century ago reached their mid-40s and then dropped dead. Visit an old cemetery, and you'll see it wasn't uncommon for our ancestors to live to ripe old ages. But you'll also find that a substantial percentage of infants, children, and childbearing women died, which brought average life expectancies down considerably.

Longevity has increased in the last 100 years largely because of measures such as sanitation, vaccinations, and antibiotics, which have helped control the infectious diseases that were often responsible for deaths of the young. With mortality rates for these populations now extremely low in the developed world, however, further improvements will have to come from extending the lives of people who have reached middle and old age. Indeed, that's been happening during the past few decades, thanks to declining death rates from heart disease, stroke, and cancer. But as Olshansky and Carnes write in their book *The Quest for Immortality*, "Adding 80 years to the life of an 80-year-old person is far more difficult than adding 80 years to the life of an infant." That requires biomedical advances to fundamentally alter the aging process—something that currently isn't possible. Based on the trends, it's reasonable to expect that improved medical and preventive care will continue allowing more and more people to make it to 90 or 100—but not to 150 or 170, as anti-aging enthusiasts predict.

Something else that's notable in the A4M response is its definition of anti-aging medicine: "the application of advanced scientific and medical technologies for the early detection, prevention, treatment, and reversal of age-related dysfunction, disorders, and diseases." In other words, minimizing the impact of age-related conditions—a worthwhile and achievable goal that's shared by many conventional health providers.

Anti-aging advocates tend to play up this definition whenever they want to make their field seem scientifically mainstream. On other occasions, however, they talk about stopping or reversing aging itself, which is an entirely different—and so far unachievable—goal. Klatz and Goldman offer up such a possibility through books with titles such as *Stopping the Clock: Dramatic Breakthroughs in Anti-Aging and Age Reversal Techniques*, which includes the A4M rallying cry, "Aging is not inevitable!"

Anti-aging doctors and clinics often cite research on the benefits of measures like exercise as evidence that aging can be slowed or reversed. Don't be fooled by this. Physical activity and other lifestyle measures may indeed help us live longer, healthier lives by reducing the risk of disability, chronic disease, and early death. But this involves preventing or delaying the signs and effects of aging—not the aging process itself. It's an important distinction that anti-aging practitioners too often fail to make.

When confronted with claims about stopping or reversing aging, we would do well to remember the words of one poster on the AARP's Internet message board: "Aging can be stopped. That is a fact! It's called death."

SUCCESSFUL AGING

Nevertheless, research does suggest a number of steps you can take to increase your chances of a long and healthy life, none of which require going to an expensive anti-aging clinic. For example, a landmark study of thousands of healthy people over 70, sponsored by the MacArthur Foundation, identified regular exercise—both aerobic and resistance training—

as "the single most important thing an older person can do to remain healthy." Other keys to "successful aging," as the researchers call it, are staying mentally active and remaining socially connected.

A study of Japanese American men found that those who in midlife were physically stronger and lean and who didn't smoke, drink alcohol in excess, or have high blood sugar or hypertension were most likely to survive to age 85 and remain healthy. A large study of centenarians and their families, led by Dr. Thomas Perls at Boston University, reveals that an ability to handle stress is another common feature of those who live exceptionally long, healthy lives.

Anti-aging doctors will tell you that by going beyond such measures and offering all kinds of tests, dietary supplements, and hormones, they're practicing "ultimate preventive medicine," as one clinic calls it. What they often won't tell you is that the science is far shakier for many of these "advanced" methods than for basic preventive steps. When forced to acknowledge the dearth of rigorous, long-term studies, they're quick to say such research will take too long to complete. "We'd have to wait," says Dr. Klatz, "until the baby boomers are dead and in the ground and worms' meat."

Certainly, this shouldn't be an excuse for not conducting randomized studies. However long they take, they're the only hope we have for getting definitive answers. In the meantime, we have to make decisions with the information that's currently available. Despite what anti-aging practitioners lead us to believe, the research as a whole fails to make a convincing case for the benefits of many of their regimens and raises troubling questions about the possible risks. Of all people, doctors who claim to be at the forefront of prevention should recognize this and lead the charge for rigorous studies that can help us make more informed decisions. As healthy skeptics, we should expect and demand nothing less.

TRUSTWORTHY SOURCES OF INFORMATION

Successful Aging by John Rowe and Robert Kahn (New York: Pantheon, 1998). Based on the findings of the MacArthur Foundation study on aging, this book explains how to avoid illness and remain active as we get older.

Living to 100: Lessons in Living to Your Maximum Potential at Any Age, by Thomas Perls and Margery Hutter Silver, with John Lauerman (New York: Basic, 1999). This book shares the lessons of the New England Centenarian Study (of which Dr. Perls is director), discussing the traits and lifestyles of those who have led long, healthy lives. It also includes a life expectancy calculator, an expanded version of which is accessible at www.livingto100.com.

The Quest for Immortality: Science at the Frontiers of Aging, by S. Jay Olshansky and Bruce Carnes (New York: Norton, 2001). In an engaging and entertaining way, this book reviews the science of aging, separating myths from facts about what it takes to live a long, healthy life.

KUDZU/Doug Marlette
© 1988 Tribune Media Services

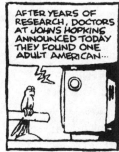

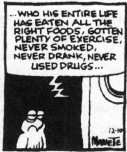

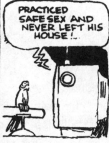

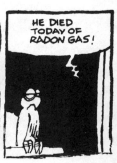

CHAPTER TEN: GUARANTEED!
OVERPROMISING ON PREVENTION

J. I. Rodale, whom we met in chapter 1, often touted his own good health as evidence for his ideas. In a June 1971 cover story in the *New York Times* magazine, which called the seemingly vigorous 72-year-old health promoter a "walking testimonial to his health theories," Rodale stated, "I'm going to live to be 100 unless I'm run down by a sugar-crazed taxi driver." (As discussed earlier, he viewed sugar as poison.)

Appearing the next day on the *Dick Cavett Show*, Rodale similarly boasted that, thanks to his regimen, "I am so healthy that I expect to live on and on." But it wasn't to be. Later in the program, as another guest was being interviewed, Rodale slumped in his chair, and his head drooped. At first, the audience laughed, thinking Rodale was pretending to fall asleep out of boredom. But Cavett quickly realized it was no joke. Two doctors rushed to the stage to administer aid, and an ambulance was called. After arriving at the hospital a short time later, Rodale was pronounced dead. He had suffered a massive heart attack.

Many wondered how this could have happened to someone so health-conscious. In a letter to the *New York Times*, one writer suggested that Rodale's death might have resulted from taking too many vitamins and not relaxing enough. Others, also implicitly blaming Rodale for his own death, expressed disappointment and even anger. Said one supporter: "Rodale has ruined the entire health-food industry by dying."

Thirteen years later, there were similar reactions when 52-year-old fitness guru and best-selling author Jim Fixx, whose promotion of the health benefits of running had helped spawn a national craze, dropped dead of a heart attack while jogging. Stunned at the news, people groped for explanations, with many recalling that Fixx had previously been overweight and a smoker and noting that he had failed to get medical checkups.

There's also the example of Dr. Lynn Smaha. A cardiologist and former president of the American Heart Association, Dr. Smaha spoke frequently about the importance of diet, exercise, and other health behaviors. To head off strokes and heart attacks, which he said were "often preventable," he urged people to improve their health habits and publicly chastised fellow doctors for not setting a better example. After exercising on a spring day in 2006, Dr. Smaha collapsed from a heart attack and died. He was 63.

Noting Smaha's passing in a blog entry titled "Dr. Lynn Allan Smaha RIP," one physician wrote: "Dr. Smaha, I'm sure, followed his own advice. . . . He did everything he recommended to others to avoid heart disease, yet he succumbed to a heart attack. If cholesterol were the cause of heart disease, if a low-fat diet were truly 'heart healthy,' if aerobic exercise kept coronary arteries supple and plaque-free, then Dr. Smaha would surely still be with us today." In other words, Dr. Smaha's untimely death had disproved everything he preached, according to this doctor, who is an advocate of a high-protein/low-carbohydrate diet. He went on to muse: "I wonder if Dr. Smaha's outcome would have been different had he followed a low-carb diet."

Underlying the reactions to these three deaths is a common misconception: that our health is entirely within our hands. If we do the right things, this thinking goes, we're virtually guaranteed good health. When someone is struck by a "preventable" illness such as heart disease, this logic may lead us to conclude that somehow it's the victim's own fault.

A major source of this misunderstanding is the very industry of which Rodale, Fixx, and Smaha were a part. These health promoters and others like them have profoundly shaped our view of health, prompting us to see it largely as a matter of individual responsibility and choice. They have sold us so vigorously—and so effectively—on the power of healthy living that we're led to have unrealistic expectations about what it will do for each of us personally.

Just because we lack complete control, however, doesn't mean that we're helpless or that our actions don't matter. What we do can have a potentially enormous impact on our health. Being a healthy skeptic requires having a sense of perspective about both the possibilities and the limits of prevention and of the advice related to it. No health regimen can guarantee that we'll "live on and on," but the right one, pursued the right way, may very well enhance the quality of our lives.

PREVENTION, PROBABILITIES, AND PROTECTIVE ILLUSIONS

Statistics reported from health studies are much like gambling odds. They express the likelihood of winning (avoiding illness) or losing (falling victim to it) among large groups of people, and they estimate how certain behaviors and other factors may change those odds. For example, men who run at least an hour a week have a 42 percent lower probability of developing heart disease than those who don't run. But running doesn't *guarantee* men won't get heart disease, just as buying multiple lottery tickets doesn't *guarantee* you'll win the jackpot. It means only that the odds may be improved.

Yet health promoters sometimes make exercise and other measures seem as though they're sure bets. Part of the problem is the imprecise use of the term "prevent." Though the word is widely used as a synonym for "reduce the risk" (as it is in this book), this meaning isn't always clear. Hearing that exercise "prevents" heart disease, we may mistakenly infer that it provides absolute protection, when in fact almost nothing we do can guarantee we'll avoid illness. Our risk may decrease—perhaps even substantially—as a result of our actions, but rarely will it be zero. Some people who exercise will develop heart disease, some nonsmokers will get lung cancer, and some who do everything right will die young.

One reason, of course, is that genetics plays a role in our susceptibility to many diseases. As the saying goes, we can't choose our parents. But the message we sometimes get from health promoters is that we can overcome our genetic predispositions if we try hard enough. For example, a billboard I used to pass daily promoted pomegranate tea with the slogan "Override your genetics." The implication of the ad was that downing this beverage could somehow help us escape our biological makeup.

Messages like this echo an axiom many health promoters are fond of reciting: "Genetics loads the gun, but lifestyle pulls the trigger." On the one hand, this metaphor is apt because it correctly reminds us that whatever our genetic makeup, there may be things we can do to help ourselves. But, on the other, it misleadingly implies that lifestyle is ultimately the determining factor—that the gun won't fire if we do all the right things. The truth is that lifestyle can indeed pull the trigger. But so can genetics.

If we believe we have the power to "override" our genes, then when something goes wrong, the tendency is to blame ourselves or others for failing to do enough. Consider, for example, the reaction when it was revealed in 2004 that former president Bill Clinton had blocked arteries and needed bypass surgery. Newspapers, television programs, and Web sites were filled with speculation about the likely culprits—his weight, his cholesterol level, his hectic work schedule, his love of cigars, and his much-parodied affinity for fast food. As discussed in chapter 6, some testing centers also pointed to his failure to get a heart scan. Even Clinton himself speculated publicly about how he might have fallen short.

In truth, the former president has a family history of heart disease, and it's impossible to know which factors played a role in his particular case. That's because epidemiology concerns probabilities in populations, not cause and effect in individuals. As a group, men who eat a diet consisting largely of red meat, French fries, refined carbs, and high-fat dairy products, for example, have a greater likelihood of developing heart disease than those who eat mainly fruits, vegetables, fish, and whole grains. But it doesn't follow that if a fast-food fanatic develops heart disease, we can be sure that his or her diet is to blame. Heart disease and other chronic conditions typically occur because of a complex interaction of genetics, environment, and lifestyle. When we try to extrapolate from population-wide risk statistics to explain individual instances of illness, we're guilty of both oversimplifying reality and misapplying epidemiology.

This way of thinking is certainly understandable, however. We tend to grasp for simple answers because of our need to explain the inexplicable and to have a sense of control over our health. In a way, it's comforting to believe that Bill Clinton's love of Big Macs did him in, because it offers reassurance that disease doesn't strike randomly and that what happened to him won't also happen to us. Psychologists call this a "protective illusion."

Health promoters have long fed this need, sometimes as a way to save face when their advice is called into question. For example, when nineteenth-century health promoter Dr. William Alcott argued that a particular diet could ward off all kinds of ailments, including flu and fever, he recognized that experience seemed to suggest otherwise. Addressing the issue in his writings, he asked rhetorically: "How could a person in perfect health, and obeying, to an iota, all the laws of health—how could he contract disease?" His answer was simple: the victims were to blame. Their prior health habits, he wrote, had "already sown the seeds of disease," and they were "almost sure to die whenever disease does attack them, simply on account of the previous abuses of their constitutions." Through such logic, Alcott reinforced people's protective illusions of control over their health while also deflecting criticism of his ideas.

Today's health promoters sometimes offer a subtler version of this reasoning in the form of "if onlys": fewer people would have heart attacks *if only* their normal cholesterol levels were even lower; fewer would develop melanoma *if only* they used sunscreen more often; fewer would die of various diseases *if only* everyone would get certain screening tests. With such assertions, health promoters imply that the problem lies with us; we need to do more, to go further, to be more diligent. The promise of whatever they're promoting isn't being fully realized, they suggest, because of our failure to comply. What health promoters should be telling us—and often don't—is that regardless of how faithfully we follow their advice, some of us will develop "preventable" illnesses through no fault of our own.

SELF-FULFILLING PROPHECIES

Understanding that prevention has limits doesn't mean we should become fatalistic about our health, however. The steps we take to stay healthy can and do matter, possibly a great deal. When people wrongly believe that disease and disability are inevitable and there's nothing they can do, it can become a self-fulfilling prophecy. One study found, for example, that those who subscribe to fatalistic beliefs such as "there's not much people can do to lower their chances of cancer" are less likely than others to exercise regularly and eat healthfully. And people who agree that "there are so many recommendations about preventing cancer, it's hard to know which ones to follow" are more likely to smoke.

So how do we sort through the countless recommendations about cancer and everything else without succumbing to the temptation just to give up and do whatever we want? Unquestionably, it can be a challenge, but following three basic rules can make the task a little easier.

1. CONSIDER THE SOURCE.

Regardless of where the advice comes from—whether news, advertisements, best-selling authors, celebrities, government officials, health groups, or consumer activists—we need to consider who's behind it and what their motives might be. As the previous chapters illustrate, determining what drives health promoters requires looking beneath the surface. For example, is that celebrity who's telling us to get tested being swayed by emotion or money rather than reason? Is that activist group issuing a scary warning to further its own agenda? Is that news organization sensationalizing a story to increase readership or ratings? Is that researcher so invested in a recommendation that he or she stubbornly sticks to it no matter what? Is that health group or government agency dumbing down advice because it assumes we can't understand nuance?

We shouldn't automatically accept advice simply because a health promoter seems, on the surface, to be trustworthy. Sources such as nonprofit groups, university scientists, and government agencies often do provide valuable and credible advice. But not always. We need to critically evaluate what they tell us just as we would the advice of anyone else.

At the same time, we shouldn't assume that someone is untrustworthy simply because they're trying to sell a product. Those with vested financial interests sometimes supply us with reliable advice that can benefit our health. If we reflexively disregard everything they tell us, we deny ourselves potentially valuable information. The idea is not to be a cynic who vilifies entire groups of health promoters; it's to be an equal-opportunity skeptic who critically analyzes all advice.

2. SCRUTINIZE THE SCIENCE.

To properly evaluate a piece of advice, it's important to understand the scientific basis for it: what kinds of supporting studies have been conducted, and how credible and relevant are they? Often, getting answers to questions such as those outlined in chapter 1 requires some digging. (The trustworthy sources listed at the end of each chapter can be good places to start.) Though all this demands some extra time and effort, the issues at stake—our health and possibly our lives—are certainly worth it.

Whether the issue is diet, sunscreen, cholesterol, hormones, or anything else, we shouldn't always expect yes or no answers from the science. Doing so sets us up for frustration and fatalism. Instead, we should be prepared to make judgment calls based on studies that may be conflicting and less than conclusive. And once we make a judgment, we should be willing to later revisit and change it if warranted. That's because research is constantly expanding our knowledge, getting us closer to the truth about how best to protect our health. Sometimes this means that an action we thought was beneficial (for example, taking beta-carotene) turns out not to be. While such changes can test our patience with scientists, they're actually a sign that science is working as intended. Think about it: the advice of pre-scientific health promoters such as Sylvester Graham rarely budged because it was based on fixed beliefs. Evidence-based advice, in contrast, is supposed to change because its foundation, scientific knowledge, is always evolving.

Dealing with information that isn't always black and white and that often changes can be maddening. But if we want science to guide our actions, we have to try to adjust how we think. And it does get easier with practice.

3. PRIORITIZE.

Not all advice is of equal importance and relevance, yet health promoters can lead us to believe otherwise by failing to provide any frame of reference. We know that smoking increases the risk of cancer, for example, but we also hear equally dire warnings about potential threats of far less magnitude and certainty such as using hair dye, eating grilled meat, and talking on cell phones. Likewise, we know that exercise decreases our risk of dying from heart disease, but we're told to embrace, with equal urgency, less proven measures such as taking antioxidants, eating walnuts, and getting heart scans.

Trying to keep up with and act on all the nuggets of advice we get can be overwhelming. And it may divert our attention from measures that really matter. To avoid this, we need to prioritize—to determine, based on the science, what's most likely to benefit us in the biggest way and stay focused on that.

The exact list of priorities will vary from person to person, depending on health status, family history, age, and other factors. But a few steps should be on everyone's list:

- Don't smoke

- Get regular physical activity

- Eat a healthful diet (heavy on fruits, vegetables, whole grains, fish, and legumes; light on refined carbs, junk food, and red meat; and with "good" fats replacing saturated and trans fats). Keep portions limited.

- Wear a seat belt

- Don't drink alcohol in excess

- Get vaccinated

- Talk to your doctor about screening tests

- Find positive ways to handle stress

One of the reasons we get frustrated with health advice and give up is that there's too much to remember: What foods have flavanols? Which ones are low on the glycemic index? Which antioxidant supplements should I take? What kinds of skillets am I supposed to avoid? How often can I use hair dye? How much DHEA should I take? But prevention doesn't have to be this complicated. By focusing on a few "big ticket" items such as those just listed, we increase the odds that we'll stick with our efforts over the long term and therefore do ourselves more good.

FINAL THOUGHTS

Amid the rampant selling of health, it's easy to lose sight of the purpose of this whole pursuit: to enhance the quality of our lives by allowing us to feel better and spend less time sick and disabled. But when we let our pursuit become a preoccupation by, for example, constantly fretting over our food or obsessing over our cholesterol levels or chasing after the secret to stopping aging, we can end up diminishing the quality of our lives. Harvard psychiatrist Arthur Barsky has noted that though we're healthier and living longer than ever, our obsession with health has paradoxically caused us greater anxiety. "The more assiduously we try to guard our good health," he wrote in his book *Worried Sick*, "the less confident and assured we become, and the less we are able to enjoy it." The late physician and author Lewis Thomas sounded a similar theme, writing that because of "propaganda" from health promoters, we are in danger of becoming "a nation of healthy hypochondriacs, living gingerly, worrying ourselves half to death."

Indeed, health promoters fuel this anxiety by constantly reminding us of all the terrible things that can befall us—heart disease, cancer, diabetes, debilitation, premature death—and telling us that we have the power, and indeed the duty, to save ourselves. We need to keep such messages in perspective, remembering that our quest for health should be about hope— hope that we are helping ourselves—not fear. We also need to be on guard against getting carried away. As the columnist George Will has written, "Health, like any wealth, can be pursued too ardently and hoarded too greedily. The result is the crabbed, sad, anxious, morally unhealthy life of a miser."

It's another reminder that, contrary to what we might believe, trying to stay healthy is not a no-lose proposition. We stand to waste money, time, and effort and possibly even cause ourselves physical or emotional harm when we follow the wrong advice or take things too far.

Nevertheless, healthful living, properly practiced, can result in a big payoff. Though there are no guarantees, taking the right steps can enhance the quality of our lives and perhaps even extend them. In the end, being a healthy skeptic comes down to maximizing your odds by figuring out which cards dealt by health promoters you should keep and which you should throw out.

Here's hoping that some of what you've read here can help you arrange a winning hand.

NOTES

All URLs were current as of January 1, 2008.

INTRODUCTION

p. 3   *"My plea is that you live health, talk health"*: Bundesen delivered this speech at the annual meeting of the American Public Health Association, October 15, 1928. For the full text, see Herman Bundesen, "Selling Health—A Vital Duty," *American Journal of Public Health* 18 (1928): 1451–1454.

p. 4   *"a few wellness entrepreneurs"*: Paul Zane Pilzer, *The Wellness Revolution: How to Make a Fortune in the Next Trillion Dollar Industry* (New York: Wiley, 2002), 198.

p. 5   *"staggering catastrophe"*: Robert Wilson, *Feminine Forever* (New York: M. Evans, 1966).

p. 6   *"There doesn't seem to be a sexy thing"*: Quoted in Amanda Spake, "The Menopausal Marketplace," *U.S. News and World Report*, November 18, 2002, 42. Spake provides an excellent overview of the hormone replacement hype.

p. 6   *funded by Premarin's manufacturer, Wyeth-Ayerst*: Information concerning the funding of Wilson's book and foundation comes from his son, Ronald Wilson. See Gina Kolata, with Melody Petersen, "Hormone Replacement Study a Shock to the Medical System," *New York Times*, July 10, 2002.

p. 6   *"The press, whether through intentional"*: Barbara Seaman, *The Greatest Experiment Ever Performed on Women: Exploding the Estrogen Myth* (New York: Hyperion, 2003), 169.

p. 6   *"years of research have painted"*: Sharon Begley, with Karen Springen, "A Clear Signal on Estrogen," *Newsweek*, June 30, 1997, 60.

p. 7   *"if there was a similar medication"*: Dr. Judith Reichman, *Today Show*, NBC
        News, transcript, September 24, 1997.

p. 7   *"It is safe today"*: Lila Nachtigall and Joan Rattner Heilman, *Estrogen: A
        Complete Guide to Menopause and Hormone Replacement Therapy*, 3rd ed. (New
        York: HarperCollins, 2000), 2–3.

p. 7   *the recipients of speaking fees, research grants, or other funding*: Sharyl Attkisson,
        "The Hormone Hype: Docs Promoting HRT Often Financially Tied to
        Drugmakers," *CBS Evening News*, November 20, 2002, www.cbsnews.com/
        stories/2002/11/20/eveningnews/main530133.shtml.

p. 7   *"my No. 1 secret"*: Lauren Hutton quoted in Joan Tarshis, "Celebrities Re-
        veal Their Secrets," *Parade*, March 19, 2000, 10–12. For more on Hutton
        and other celebrities involved in marketing HRT, see Ray Moynihan and
        Alan Cassels, *Selling Sickness: How the World's Biggest Pharmaceutical Compa-
        nies Are Turning Us All into Patients* (New York: Nation Books, 2005), 41–60.

p. 7   *Women's Health Initiative*: National Institutes of Health, National Heart,
        Lung, and Blood Institute, "NHLBI Stops Trial of Estrogen plus Progestin
        due to Increased Breast Cancer Risk, Lack of Overall Benefit," news
        release, July 9, 2002, www.nhlbi.nih.gov/new/press/02-07-09.htm. The re-
        search findings are reported in Writing Group for the Women's Health Ini-
        tiative Randomized Controlled Trial, "Risks and Benefits of Estrogen plus
        Progestin in Healthy Postmenopausal Women: Principal Results from the
        Women's Health Initiative Randomized Controlled Trial," *Journal of the
        American Medical Association* 288 (2002): 321–333. The findings on demen-
        tia are reported in Stephen Rapp et al., "Effect of Estrogen plus Progestin
        on Global Cognitive Function in Postmenopausal Women," *Journal of the
        American Medical Association* 289 (2003): 2663–2672. For a good summary
        of the research and what it means for women, see "Facts about Menopausal
        Hormone Therapy," available at www.nhlbi.nih.gov/health/women/pht
        _facts.pdf.

p. 8   *"we made observations and hypotheses"*: Susan Love, "Preventive Medicine,
        Properly Practiced," *New York Times*, July 16, 2002.

p. 8   *"a triumph of marketing over science"*: Cynthia Pearson quoted in "Response
        to the Announcement that Health Risks Outweigh Benefits for Combined
        Estrogen plus Progestin," statement from the National Women's Health
        Network, July 2002.

p. 11   *"Cynicism is much easier than skepticism"*: Marcia Angell, *Science on Trial: The
        Clash of Medical Evidence and the Law in the Breast Implant Case* (New York:
        Norton, 1996), 158.

p. 11   *one-third of all U.S. deaths*: Centers for Disease Control and Prevention, *The
        Power of Prevention: Reducing the Health and Economic Burden of Chronic Dis-
        ease, 2003*, www.cdc.gov/nccdphp/publications/PowerOfPrevention.

1. SAYS WHO?

In addition to the specific citations below, sources for this chapter include the following works: L. Margaret Barnett, "The Impact of 'Fletcherism' on the Food Policies of Herbert Hoover during World War I," *Bulletin of the History of Medicine* 66 (1992): 234–259; L. Hill Curth, "Lessons from the Past: Preventive Medicine in Early Modern England," *Medical Humanities* 29 (2003): 16–20; Ronald Deutsch, *The Nuts among the Berries: An Exposé of America's Food Fads* (New York: Ballantine, 1967); Ruth Clifford Engs, *Clean Living Movements: American Cycles of Health Reform* (Westport, Conn.: Praeger, 2000); Michael Goldstein, *The Health Movement: Promoting Fitness in America* (New York: Twayne, 1992); Anita Guerrini, *Obesity and Depression in the Enlightenment: The Life and Times of George Cheyne* (Norman: University of Oklahoma Press, 2000); Charles Hennekens and Julie Buring, *Epidemiology in Medicine* (Boston: Little, Brown, 1987); Thomas Horrocks, "'The Poor Man's Riches, The Poor Man's Bliss': Regimen, Reform, and the *Journal of Health*, 1829–1933," *Proceedings of the American Philosophical Society* 139 (1995): 115–134; Richard Schwarz, *John Harvey Kellogg, MD* (Nashville: Southern Publishing Association, 1970).

p. 13   *The Road to Wellville:* The 1994 movie, directed by Alan Parker, was based on T. Coraghessan Boyle's novel of the same name, published by Viking in 1993.

p. 13   *"my own stools":* The comment about odor was actually made by health promoter Horace Fletcher, who, in contrast, bragged about the smallness of his stools. See James Whorton, *Inner Hygiene: Constipation and the Pursuit of Health in Modern Society* (New York: Oxford University Press, 2000), 160–161.

p. 14   *"there are more than 900 studies":* Kevin Trudeau, *Natural Cures "They" Don't Want You to Know About* (Elk Grove Village, Ill.: Alliance Publishing, 2004), 319.

p. 15   *"If men would but observe the golden mean":* George Cheyne, *An Essay of Health and Long Life* (London: George Strahan, 1745), 230–231. Quoting Cheyne here and elsewhere, I have modernized spelling and capitalization in order to make the passages more readable.

p. 15   *"I have consulted nothing":* Ibid., xvi.

p. 16   *"the great secret of health and long life":* Ibid., 230.

p. 16   *"shaking the whole machine":* Ibid., 94–95.

p. 16   *"infinite experiment":* George Cheyne quoted in Steven Shapin, "Trusting George Cheyne: Scientific Expertise, Common Sense, and Moral Authority in Early Eighteenth-Century Dietetic Medicine," *Bulletin of the History of Medicine* 77 (2003): 263–297.

p. 16   *"air, food, exercise":* Quoted in Stephen Nissenbaum, *Sex, Diet, and Debility in Jacksonian America: Sylvester Graham and Health Reform* (Westport, Conn.: Greenwood Press, 1980), 76. This statement of purpose was included in a notice printed at the end of each issue of the journal.

p. 17   *"only competent judge"*: Quoted in Harvey Green, *Fit for America: Health, Fitness, Sport, and American Society* (New York: Pantheon, 1986), 13.

p. 17   *"all medicine, as such, is itself an evil"*: Sylvester Graham quoted in Ronald Numbers, *Prophetess of Health: A Study of Ellen G. White* (New York: Harper and Row, 1976), 54.

p. 17   *"morally binding duty"*: Quoted in James Whorton, *Crusaders for Fitness: The History of American Health Reformers* (Princeton, N.J.: Princeton University Press, 1982), 60.

p. 18   *"Am I at fault"*: William Alcott, *The Physiology of Marriage* (Boston: Jewett, 1855), 118–119.

p. 18   *"It is much easier"*: William Alcott, *Forty Years in the Wilderness of Pills and Powders* (Boston: Jewett, 1859), 97–98.

p. 19   *"independent of books"*: Ellen White quoted in Numbers, *Prophetess of Health*, 84.

p. 19   *she frequently lifted passages almost verbatim:* Ibid., 162–167.

p. 20   *"the most formidable reformer"*: Whorton, *Inner Hygiene*, 182.

p. 21   *"the most dangerous of all sexual abuses"*: John Harvey Kellogg, *Plain Facts for Old and Young* (New York: Arno, 1974), 231. This work was first published in 1877 under the title *Plain Facts about Sexual Life*. Kellogg railed against masturbation in *Plain Facts* for nearly 100 pages—more space than he devoted to any other topic in the book.

p. 21   *"neither the plague, nor war"*: Ibid., 233.

p. 21   *Kellogg's masturbation remedies for males and females:* Ibid., 295–296.

p. 21   *"pretentious quacks"*: Ibid., 326.

p. 22   *"had done more to help suffering humanity"*: John Harvey Kellogg quoted in Whorton, *Crusaders for Fitness*, 205.

p. 22   *"with greater ease"*: Ibid., 185.

p. 22   *"the science of guessing"*: "Medicine, The Science of Guessing" was a chapter title in Macfadden's *Encyclopedia of Physical Culture*. See William Hunt, *Body Love: The Amazing Career of Bernarr Macfadden* (Bowling Green, Ohio: Bowling Green State University Popular Press, 1989), 68.

p. 22   *"to the ignorance of the distant past"*: Robert Ernst, *Weakness Is a Crime: The Life of Bernarr Macfadden* (Syracuse, N.Y.: Syracuse University Press, 1991), 22.

p. 23   *"that French quack"*: Hunt, *Body Love*, 58.

p. 24   *enthusiastic blessing to "natural" food supplements:* Carlton Jackson, *J. I. Rodale: Apostle of Nonconformity* (New York: Pyramid, 1974), 131.

p. 24   *"Happy People Rarely Get Cancer"*: This article appeared in *Prevention* mag-

azine in November 1966. Rodale's book of the same name was published by
Rodale Press in 1970.

p. 25   *"fanciful interpretation of selected medical literature":* Harriet Hall and Stephen
Barrett, "A Skeptical View of the Perricone Prescription," www.quackwatch
.org/11Ind/perricone.html.

p. 26   *Seven Countries Study:* For more on the research and the celebrated scientist
Ancel Keys, who spearheaded it, see www.epi.umn.edu/research/7countries/
overview.shtm.

p. 27   *bladder cancer and hair dye:* See, for example, Manuela Gago-Dominguez et
al., "Use of Permanent Hair Dyes and Bladder-Cancer Risk," *International
Journal of Cancer* 91 (2001): 575–579.

p. 27   *the ongoing Framingham Heart Study:* For an overview of this study, see
www.nhlbi.nih.gov/about/framingham.

p. 29   *male smokers are 23 times more likely:* American Cancer Society, "Smoking
and Cancer Mortality Table," www.cancer.org/docroot/PED/content/PED
_10_2X_Smoking_and_Cancer_Mortality_Table.asp.

p. 29   *association between breast cancer and alcohol consumption:* Pamela Horn-Ross et
al., "Patterns of Alcohol Consumption and Breast Cancer Risk in the California Teachers Cohort Study," *Cancer Epidemiology, Biomarkers and Prevention* 13 (2004): 405–411.

p. 31   *Studies are sometimes presented at scientific conferences:* See Lisa Schwartz,
Steven Woloshin, and Linda Baczek, "Media Coverage of Scientific Meetings: Too Much, Too Soon?" *Journal of the American Medical Association* 287
(2002): 2859–2863.

2. THE NEWS MEDIA

p. 36   *certain broad categories of foods . . . may be beneficial:* See, for example, Feng
He, Caryl Nowson, and Graham MacGregor, "Fruit and Vegetable Con-
sumption and Stroke: Meta-analysis of Cohort Studies," *Lancet* 367 (2006):
320–326; Teresa Fung et al., "Dietary Patterns and the Risk of Coronary
Heart Disease in Women," *Archives of Internal Medicine* 161 (2001): 1857–
1862; Raphaelle Varraso et al., "Prospective Study of Dietary Patterns and
Chronic Obstructive Pulmonary Disease among U.S. Men," *Thorax* 62
(2007): 786–791.

p. 36   *lycopene research:* Edward Giovannucci, "Tomato Products, Lycopene, and
Prostate Cancer: A Review of the Epidemiological Literature," *Journal of
Nutrition* 135 (2005): 2030S–2031S. For examples of studies finding no
association, see Victoria Kirsch et al., "A Prospective Study of Lycopene
and Tomato Product Intake and Risk of Prostate Cancer," *Cancer Epidemiology, Biomarkers and Prevention* 15 (2006): 92–98; and Ulrike Peters et al.,
"Serum Lycopene, Other Carotenoids, and Prostate Cancer Risk: A Nested

Case-Control Study in the Prostate, Lung, Colorectal, and Ovarian Cancer Screening Trial," *Cancer Epidemiology, Biomarkers and Prevention* 16 (2007): 962–968.

p. 37   *"an easy and tasty way"*: H.J. Heinz Company, "Making Small Dietary Changes Can Have a Big Impact on Health," news release, October 24, 2005.

p. 38   *The headlines are attention-grabbing*: "Beans and Soy May Help Prevent Lung Cancer," UPI, October 3, 2005; "Onions Could Be Good for the Bones," *Seattle Post-Intelligencer*, April 7, 2005; "Raisins May Help Fight Cavities," WebMD, June 8, 2005, www.webmd.com/food-recipes/news/20050608/raisins-may-help-fight-cavities; "Sauerkraut Packed with Cancer-Fighting Compounds," Reuters Health, October 21, 2002; "Alfalfa Could Fight Vision Loss," *Saint Paul Pioneer Press*, December 22, 2005.

p. 39   *"You'd have to be a fool"*: Michael Zemel, University of Tennessee, quoted in "Dairy Weight-Loss Claims Prompt Lawsuits," *Washington Post*, June 29, 2005.

p. 39   *financial ties to olestra's manufacturer*: Jane Levine et al., "Authors' Financial Relationships with the Food and Beverage Industry and Their Published Positions on the Fat Substitute Olestra," *American Journal of Public Health* 93 (2003): 664–669.

p. 39   *an analysis of studies on soft drinks, juices, and milk*: Lenard Lesser et al., "Relationship between Funding Source and Conclusion among Nutrition-Related Scientific Articles," *PLoS Medicine* 4 (2007): e5, http://medicine.plosjournals.org/perlserv/?request=get-document&doi=10.1371/journal.pmed.0040005.

p. 39   *"it seems counter-intuitive"*: Marion Nestle, "Food Company Sponsorship of Nutrition Research and Professional Activities: A Conflict of Interest?" *Public Health Nutrition* 4 (2001): 1015–1022.

p. 39   *"when the negotiations come down to the wire"*: Martijn Katan, "Does Industry Sponsorship Undermine the Integrity of Nutrition Research?" *PLoS Medicine* 4 (2007): e6, http://medicine.plosjournals.org/perlserv/?request=get-document&doi=10.1371/journal.pmed.0040006.

p. 41   *they continue to be widely used by stations*: Diane Farsetta and Daniel Price, "Fake TV News: Widespread and Undisclosed," Center for Media and Democracy, April 6, 2006, www.prwatch.org/fakenews/execsummary.

p. 42   *eating nuts and a lower risk of heart disease*: See, for example, Christine Albert et al., "Nut Consumption and Decreased Risk of Sudden Cardiac Death in the Physicians' Health Study," *Archives of Internal Medicine* 162 (2002): 1382–1387; Frank Hu et al., "Frequent Nut Consumption and Risk of Coronary Heart Disease in Women: Prospective Cohort Study," *British Medical Journal* 317 (1998): 1341–1345; Frank Hu and Meir Stampfer,

"Nut Consumption and Risk of Coronary Heart Disease: A Review of Epidemiologic Evidence," *Current Atherosclerosis Reports* 1 (1999): 204–209.

p. 42   *"21st Century 'Super Food'"*: This description and the "packed with nutrients" reference come from California Walnut Commission, "California Walnuts Health Research Update," October 2006, 3, www.walnuts.org/pdfs/health/WalnutsHealthResearchUpdateOctober2006.pdf. The "essential food for health" slogan is prominently displayed on the commission's Web site, www.walnuts.org.

p. 43   *effects of a diet relatively high in ALA:* Guixiang Zhao et al., "Dietary Alpha-Linolenic Acid Reduces Inflammatory and Lipid Cardiovascular Risk Factors in Hypercholesterolemic Men and Women," *Journal of Nutrition* 134 (2004): 2991–2997.

p. 43   *"New Proof"*: California Walnut Commission, "New Proof: Walnuts Show Multiple New Heart Health Benefits," press release, November 8, 2004, www.walnutinfo.com/media/releases/proof.html. The press release includes a link to a Penn State release that does mention flaxseed oil and discloses the funding source.

p. 43   *benefits of omega-3 fats in fish:* See, for example, Charles Harper and Terry Jacobson, "Usefulness of Omega-3 Fatty Acids and the Prevention of Coronary Heart Disease," *American Journal of Cardiology* 96 (2005): 1521–1529.

p. 43   *ALA and advanced prostate cancer:* Michael Leitzmann et al., "Dietary Intake of n-3 and n-6 Fatty Acids and the Risk of Prostate Cancer," *American Journal of Clinical Nutrition* 80 (2004): 204–216.

p. 43   *"By now, you've likely heard"*: "Walnuts Are Heart Smart," WebMD, November 11, 2004, www.webmd.com/heart-disease/news/20041110/walnuts-are-heart-smart.

p. 43   *"Experts say a one-ounce serving of walnuts"*: *Health* magazine, May 2005, 180.

p. 44   *"High fish consumption"*: "Walnuts Taste Good, and Still Good for You," *Modesto Bee*, January 1, 2005.

p. 44   *walnuts were analyzed for their levels of melatonin:* Russel Reiter, L. C. Manchester, and Dun-Xian Tan, "Melatonin in Walnuts: Influence on Levels of Melatonin and Total Antioxidant Capacity of Blood," *Nutrition* 21 (2005): 920–924.

p. 44   *no long-term human trials proving that melatonin prevents disease:* For a thorough review of the evidence regarding melatonin's many proposed uses, see the National Standard database of supplements, available on the Mayo Clinic's Web site at www.mayoclinic.com/health/melatonin/NS_patient-melatonin.

p. 44   *overblown assertion in a press release headline:* California Walnut Commission,

"New Study Shows Melatonin in Walnuts Protective against Cancer and Heart Disease," press release, September 13, 2005, www.walnutinfo.com/health/melatonin.html. An accompanying press release from the University of Texas did disclose the funding source but did not mention that the study had been conducted on rats.

p. 44   *A video news release from the walnut industry:* VNR produced and distributed by News Broadcast Network for Torme Lauricella Public Relations, whose client is the California Walnut Commission; released September 14, 2005. The quoted statements are sound bites provided in addition to the prepackaged news report.

p. 45   *"You don't want to bite the hand":* telephone interview, February 27, 2007.

p. 46   *Some epidemiological studies:* Examples of research on flavanol (an alternate spelling is flavonol) include R. R. Huxley and H. A. Neil, "The Relation between Dietary Flavonol Intake and Coronary Heart Disease Mortality: A Meta-Analysis of Prospective Cohort Studies," *European Journal of Clinical Nutrition* 57 (2003): 904–908; Jennifer Lin et al., "Dietary Intakes of Flavonols and Flavones and Coronary Heart Disease in U.S. Women," *American Journal of Epidemiology* 165 (2007): 1305–1313; Eric Rimm et al., "Relation between Intake of Flavonoids and Risk for Coronary Heart Disease in Male Health Professionals," *Annals of Internal Medicine* 125 (1996): 384–389.

p. 46   *chocolate-specific research:* For a review of the evidence, see Eric Ding et al., "Chocolate and Prevention of Cardiovascular Disease: A Systematic Review," *Nutrition and Metabolism* 3 (2006): 2, www.nutritionandmetabolism .com/content/3/1/2.

p. 46   *it's not known whether the effects of chocolate are long-lasting:* One cohort study did find that subjects who consumed the most cocoa had a lower death rate from cardiovascular disease and from all causes than those who ate the least cocoa. But the researchers noted that "confirmation by other observational and experimental studies is needed." See Brian Buijsse et al., "Cocoa Intake, Blood Pressure, and Cardiovascular Mortality," *Archives of Internal Medicine* 166 (2006): 411–417.

p. 46   *a study in the journal* Hypertension: Davide Grassi et al., "Cocoa Reduces Blood Pressure and Insulin Resistance and Improves Endothelium-Dependent Vasodilation in Hypertensives," *Hypertension* 46 (2005): 398–405.

p. 46   *Mars jumped on the findings:* Mars Inc., "New Study Offers More Support for Potential Heart Health Benefits of Cocoa Flavanols," press release, July 18, 2005.

p. 47   *The American Heart Association issued its own:* American Heart Association, "Dark Chocolate May Reduce Blood Pressure, Improve Insulin Resistance," press release, July 19, 2005, www.americanheart.org/presenter.jhtml ?identifier=3032114.

p. 47   *"not saying that chocolate is now a health food"*: Jeffrey Blumberg of Tufts University quoted in "Dark Chocolate: It's Not a Health Food, But . . . ," *New York Times*, July 19, 2005.

p. 47   *"For those with hypertension, a daily dose of dark chocolate"*: "Sweet Treatment for High Blood Pressure," Knight Ridder News Service, August 9, 2005.

p. 47   *"It's another excuse to indulge your sweet tooth"*: KSDK, St. Louis, 10 P.M. news program, July 18, 2005.

p. 47   *"If you needed another reason"*: WJW, Cleveland, 8 A.M. news program, July 20, 2005.

p. 48   *"There is more conclusive evidence chocolate is good for you"*: KRCG, Jefferson City, Missouri, 5 P.M. news program, July 20, 2005.

p. 48   *"A great excuse to eat some chocolate"*: KVUE, Austin, 7 A.M. news program, July 23, 2005.

p. 49   *"definitive new research review"*: National Dairy Council, "Definitive New Research Review Sets the Record Straight about Dairy," press release, April 1, 2000. The study to which it refers is Robert Heaney, "Calcium, Dairy Products, and Osteoporosis," *Journal of the American College of Nutrition* 19 (2000): 83S–99S.

p. 49   *a recipient of dairy industry funding*: For a partial list of funding received by Heaney and other researchers, see the Integrity in Science Database (www .cspinet.org/integrity) maintained by the Center for Science in the Public Interest.

p. 49   *the evidence is mixed regarding milk's effect on bones*: See, for example, Heidi Kalkwarf, Jane Khoury, and Bruce Lanphear, "Milk Intake during Childhood and Adolescence, Adult Bone Density, and Osteoporotic Fractures in U.S. Women," *American Journal of Clinical Nutrition* 77 (2003): 257–265; Diane Feskanich, Walter Willett, and Graham Colditz, "Calcium, Vitamin D, Milk Consumption, and Hip Fractures: A Prospective Study among Postmenopausal Women," *American Journal of Clinical Nutrition* 77 (2003): 504–511.

p. 49   *"most studies of dairy food intake"*: Roland Weinsier and Carlos Krumdieck, "Dairy Foods and Bone Health: Examination of the Evidence," *American Journal of Clinical Nutrition* 72 (2000): 681–689.

p. 49   *in countries such as China and Japan*: See D. Mark Hegsted, "Fractures, Calcium, and the Modern Diet," *American Journal of Clinical Nutrition* 74 (2001): 571–573.

p. 50   *"selling the science"*: "Healthy Weight with Dairy," marketing plan overview by the Milk Processor Education Program, www.idfa.org/meetings/presentations/zaborsky202803.pdf.

p. 50   *dairy industry forced to discontinue effort*: Kim Severson, "Dairy Council to End Ad Campaign That Linked Drinking Milk with Weight Loss," *New York Times*, May 11, 2007, www.nytimes.com/2007/05/11/us/11milk.html.

p. 50   *small, short-term human experiments conducted by Michael Zemel:* Michael
        Zemel et al., "Calcium and Dairy Acceleration of Weight and Fat Loss dur-
        ing Energy Restriction in Obese Adults," *Obesity Research* 12 (2004): 582–
        590; Michael Zemel et al., "Dairy Augmentation of Total and Central Fat
        Loss in Obese Subjects," *International Journal of Obesity* 29 (2005): 391–397;
        Michael Zemel et al., "Effects of Calcium and Dairy on Body Composition
        and Weight Loss in African-American Adults," *Obesity Research* 13 (2005):
        1218–1225.

p. 50   *"proven premise" of Zemel's book:* Michael Zemel and Bill Gottlieb, *The Cal-
        cium Key: The Revolutionary Diet Discovery That Will Help You Lose Weight
        Faster* (New York: Wiley, 2003).

p. 50   *Similar studies by other investigators have found no evidence:* Jean Harvey-
        Berino et al., "The Impact of Calcium and Dairy Product Consumption on
        Weight Loss," *Obesity Research* 13 (2005): 1720–1726; Jane Bowen, Manny
        Noakes, and Peter Clifton, "Effect of Calcium and Dairy Foods in High-
        Protein, Energy-Restricted Diets on Weight Loss and Metabolic Parame-
        ters in Overweight Adults," *International Journal of Obesity* 29 (2005): 957–
        965; Catherine Berkey et al., "Milk, Dairy Fat, Dietary Calcium, and
        Weight Gain: A Longitudinal Study of Adolescents," *Archives of Pediatrics
        and Adolescent Medicine* 159 (2005): 543–550.

p. 51   *his findings apply only to overweight people:* David Schardt, "Milking the
        Data," *Nutrition Action Healthletter,* September 2005, www.cspinet.org/nah/
        09_05/milking.pdf.

p. 51   *the dairy industry's ads:* April Hermstad, "A Content Analysis of the 'Milk
        Your Diet, Lose Weight!' Campaign and an Evaluation of the Supporting
        Science," unpublished, May 2006.

p. 51   *"Got milk? If you want to lose weight":* Kristi Gustafson, "Dairy Calcium
        May Aid Weight Loss and Burn Fat," (Florida) *Sun-Sentinel,* September 30,
        2004.

p. 51   *"It's not just for strong bones and healthy muscles":* Joseph Gidjunis, "Behold
        the Power of Dairy," (Mississippi) *Sun Herald,* May 17, 2004.

p. 51   *"Milk is a natural weight-loss food":* Nate Millado, "15 Things You Need to
        Know about Milk," *Men's Fitness* magazine, March 2004.

p. 51   *A video news release from the dairy industry:* Accessed through www.national
        dairycouncil.org, April 15, 2007. The VNR is no longer available on the site.

p. 52   *one news director in Cincinnati:* Blog entry at www.allensalkin.com, April 23,
        2004; no longer available.

p. 52   *possible increased risk of prostate and ovarian cancer:* See, for example, Pana-
        giota Mitrou et al., "A Prospective Study of Dietary Calcium, Dairy Prod-
        ucts, and Prostate Cancer Risk," *International Journal of Cancer* 120 (2007):
        2466–2473; Xiang Gao, Michael LaValley, and Katherine Tucker, "Pros-

pective Studies of Dairy and Calcium Intakes and Prostate Cancer Risk: A Meta-analysis," *Journal of the National Cancer Institute* 97 (2005): 1768–1777; Susanna Larsson, Nicola Orsini, and Alicja Wolk, "Milk, Milk Products, and Lactose Intake and Ovarian Cancer Risk: A Meta-analysis of Epidemiological Studies," *International Journal of Cancer* 118 (2006): 431–441; Jeanine Genkinger et al., "Dairy Products and Ovarian Cancer: A Pooled Analysis of 12 Cohort Studies," *Cancer Epidemiology, Biomarkers and Prevention* 15 (2006): 364–372.

p. 52   *more permissive FDA rules:* For a description of the rules regarding various types of claims, see "Claims That Can Be Made for Conventional Foods and Dietary Supplements," www.cfsan.fda.gov/~dms/hclaims.html. For a list of approved qualified claims, see "Qualified Health Claims Subject to Enforcement Discretion," www.cfsan.fda.gov/~dms/qhc-sum.html.

p. 53   *equivocal claim for tomatoes:* For the FDA's assessment of the science and its rationale for allowing this claim, see Claudine Kavanaugh, Paula Trumbo, and Kathleen Ellwood, "The U.S. Food and Drug Administration's Evidence-Based Review for Qualified Health Claims: Tomatoes, Lycopene, and Cancer," *Journal of the National Cancer Institute* 99 (2007): 1074–1085.

p. 53   *An FDA study on how consumers perceive food claims:* Brenda Derby and Alan Levy, "Effects of Strength of Science Disclaimers on the Communication Impacts of Health Claims," Working Paper no. 1, Office of Regulations and Policy, Center for Food Safety and Applied Nutrition, U.S. Food and Drug Administration, September 2005, www.fda.gov/OHRMS/dockets/dockets/03N0496/03N-0496-rpt0001.pdf.

3. DIET BOOKS

p. 57   *"extraordinarily healthy cardiovascular system":* "Statement on the Status of Dr. Robert C. Atkins' Health from Dr. Atkins and from the Chief Executive Officer/President of the Atkins Companies," April 25, 2002.

p. 57   *"in no way related to diet":* Ibid.

p. 58   *"private and of no concern or relevance":* Statement by Veronica Atkins, February 9, 2004, http://usatoday.com/news/health/2004-02-10-atkins-statements_x.htm.

p. 59   *the evidence was "overwhelming":* Robert Atkins, *Crossfire*, CNN, transcript, May 30, 2000.

p. 59   *"just absolutely amazed by the results":* Arthur Agatston, *Dateline NBC*, NBC News, transcript, August 15, 2003.

p. 59   *"I've had people lose 100, 150, 200, 250 pounds":* Suzanne Somers, *Today Show*, NBC News, transcript, April 17, 2001.

p. 59   *"you can't gain weight":* Suzanne Somers, *Today Show*, NBC News, transcript, January 6, 2003.

p. 59   *"By eliminating sugar and not eating fat and carbohydrate together":* Suzanne
Somers, *CNN Saturday Morning,* CNN, transcript, August 31, 2002.

p. 59   *randomized trial studying four diets:* Michael Dansinger et al., "Comparison
of the Atkins, Ornish, Weight Watchers, and Zone Diets for Weight Loss
and Heart Disease Risk Reduction: A Randomized Trial," *Journal of the
American Medical Association* 293 (2005): 43–53.

p. 60   *Another diet-comparison trial published in* JAMA: Christopher Gardner et al.,
"Comparison of the Atkins, Zone, Ornish, and LEARN Diets for Change
in Weight and Related Risk Factors among Overweight Premenopausal
Women," *Journal of the American Medical Association* 297 (2007): 969–977.

p. 60   *in the short term . . . low-carb diets like Atkins result in greater weight loss:* Gary
Foster et al., "A Randomized Trial of a Low-Carbohydrate Diet for Obe-
sity," *New England Journal of Medicine* 348 (2003): 2082–2090; Frederick
Samaha et al., "A Low-Carbohydrate as Compared with a Low-Fat Diet in
Severe Obesity," *New England Journal of Medicine* 348 (2003): 2074–2081;
Linda Stern et al., "The Effects of Low-Carbohydrate versus Conventional
Weight Loss Diets in Severely Obese Adults: One-Year Follow-Up of a
Randomized Trial," *Annals of Internal Medicine* 140 (2004): 778–785.

p. 60   *Cochrane Collaboration review of research:* Sandi Pirozzo et al., "Advice on
Low-Fat Diets for Obesity," *Cochrane Database of Systematic Reviews* 2 (2002),
www.mrw.interscience.wiley.com/cochrane/clsysrev/articles/CD003640/
frame.html.

p. 60   *the Women's Health Initiative study:* Barbara Howard et al., "Low-Fat Dietary
Pattern and Weight Change over 7 Years: The Women's Health Initiative
Dietary Modification Trial," *Journal of the American Medical Association* 295
(2006): 39–49.

p. 60   Seinfeld *episode:* "The Non-Fat Yogurt," *Seinfeld,* NBC, episode 7, season
5, originally aired in November 1993.

p. 61   *our total calorie intake went up:* Centers for Disease Control and Prevention,
"Trends in Intake of Energy and Macronutrients, United States, 1971–
2000," *Morbidity and Mortality Weekly Report* 53 (2004): 80–82.

p. 61   *95 percent eventually regaining lost weight:* Matthew Kramer et al., "Long-
Term Follow-Up of Behavioral Treatment for Obesity: Patterns of Weight
Regain among Men and Women," *International Journal of Obesity* 13 (1989):
123–136.

p. 62   *"You will substantially increase your odds of living long and well":* Arthur Agatston, *The South Beach Diet* (New York: St. Martin's Press, 2003), 5.

p. 62   *"You will achieve good health":* Robert Atkins, *The Atkins New Diet Revolution*
(New York: HarperCollins, 2002), 10.

p. 62   *"Most people find they feel so much better":* Dean Ornish, *Crossfire,* CNN,
transcript, May 30, 2000.

p. 62   *low-carb diets can have a beneficial effect:* Alain Nordmann et al., "Effects of
         Low-Carbohydrate vs. Low-Fat Diets on Weight Loss and Cardiovascular
         Risk Factors: A Meta-Analysis of Randomized Controlled Trials," *Archives
         of Internal Medicine* 166 (2006): 285–293; Samaha et al., "A Low-Carbohy-
         drate as Compared with a Low-Fat Diet."

p. 62   *can cause constipation, headaches, and fatigue:* Arne Astrup, Thomas Larsen,
         and Angela Harper, "Atkins and Other Low-Carbohydrate Diets: Hoax or
         an Effective Tool for Weight Loss?" *Lancet* 364 (2004): 897–899; Allen
         Last and Stephen Wilson, "Low Carbohydrate Diets," *American Family
         Physician* 73 (2006): 1942–1948.

p. 63   *fat-restricted diet may reduce cholesterol:* Nordmann et al., "Effects of Low-
         Carbohydrate vs. Low-Fat Diets."

p. 63   *research suggests that limiting saturated and trans fats:* Frank Hu, JoAnn Man-
         son, and Walter Willett, "Types of Dietary Fat and Risk of Coronary Heart
         Disease: A Critical Review," *Journal of the American College of Nutrition* 20
         (2001): 5–19.

p. 63   *reducing total fat doesn't appear to lower the risk:* Barbara Howard et al., "Low-
         Fat Dietary Pattern and Risk of Cardiovascular Disease: The Women's
         Health Initiative Randomized Controlled Dietary Modification Trial,"
         Journal of the American Medical Association 295 (2006): 655–666; Shirley
         Beresford et al., "Low-Fat Dietary Pattern and Risk of Colorectal Cancer:
         The Women's Health Initiative Randomized Controlled Dietary Modifica-
         tion Trial," *Journal of the American Medical Association* 295 (2006): 643–654;
         Ross Prentice et al., "Low-Fat Dietary Pattern and Risk of Invasive Breast
         Cancer: The Women's Health Initiative Randomized Controlled Dietary
         Modification Trial," *Journal of the American Medical Association* 295 (2006):
         629–642.

p. 63   *an extremely low-fat diet can have a negative impact:* Alice Lichtenstein and
         Linda Van Horn, "Very Low Fat Diets," *Circulation* 98 (1998): 935–939.

p. 63   *Ornish study:* Dean Ornish et al., "Intensive Lifestyle Changes for Reversal
         of Coronary Heart Disease," *Journal of the American Medical Association* 280
         (1998): 2001–2007.

p. 64   *positive effects of weight loss in people who are obese:* Samuel Klein et al., "Clin-
         ical Implications of Obesity with Specific Focus on Cardiovascular Disease:
         A Statement for Professionals from the American Heart Association Coun-
         cil on Nutrition, Physical Activity, and Metabolism," *Circulation* 110 (2004):
         2952–2967; Lars Sjostrom et al., "Lifestyle, Diabetes, and Cardiovascular
         Risk Factors 10 Years after Bariatric Surgery," *New England Journal of Med-
         icine* 351 (2004): 2683–2693; Krista Haines et al., "Objective Evidence That
         Bariatric Surgery Improves Obesity-Related Obstructive Sleep Apnea,"
         Surgery 141 (2007): 354–358.

p. 64   *losing weight would allow you to live longer:* See, for example, Lars Sjostrom et al., "Effects of Bariatric Surgery on Mortality in Swedish Obese Subjects," *New England Journal of Medicine* 357 (2007): 741–752; Edward Gregg et al., "Intentional Weight Loss and Death in Overweight and Obese U.S. Adults 35 Years of Age and Older," *Annals of Internal Medicine* 138 (2003): 383–389.

p. 64   *a cohort study of Harvard alumni:* I-Min Lee and Ralph Paffenbarger, "Change in Body Weight and Longevity," *Journal of the American Medical Association* 268 (1992): 2045–2049.

p. 64   *an Israeli cohort study:* Shlomit Yaari and Uri Goldbourt, "Voluntary and Involuntary Weight Loss: Associations with Long Term Mortality in 9,228 Middle-Aged and Elderly Men," *American Journal of Epidemiology* 148 (1998): 546–555.

p. 64   *a CDC cohort study:* Elsie Pamuk et al., "Weight Loss and Mortality in a National Cohort of Adults, 1971–1987," *American Journal of Epidemiology* 136 (1992): 686–697.

p. 64   *Finnish Twin Cohort study:* Thorkild Sørensen et al., "Intention to Lose Weight, Weight Changes, and 18-y Mortality in Overweight Individuals without Co-morbidities," *PLoS Medicine* 2 (2005): e17, http://medicine .plosjournals.org/perlserv/?request=get-document&doi=10.1371/journal .pmed.0020171.

p. 65   *other cohort studies of intentional weight loss:* See, for example, David Williamson et al., "Prospective Study of Intentional Weight Loss and Mortality in Never-Smoking Overweight U.S. White Women Aged 40–64 Years," *American Journal of Epidemiology* 141 (1995): 1128–1141; David Williamson et al., "Prospective Study of Intentional Weight Loss and Mortality in Overweight White Men Aged 40–64 Years," *American Journal of Epidemiology* 149 (1999): 491–503; David Williamson et al., "Intentional Weight Loss and Mortality among Overweight Individuals with Diabetes," *Diabetes Care* 23 (2000): 1499–1504; Simone French et al., "Prospective Study of Intentionality of Weight Loss and Mortality in Older Women: The Iowa Women's Health Study," *American Journal of Epidemiology* 149 (1999): 504–514.

p. 65   *yo-yo dieting:* Aaron Folsom et al., "Weight Variability and Mortality: The Iowa Women's Health Study," *International Journal of Obesity and Related Metabolic Disorders* 20 (1996): 704–709; Simone French et al., "Weight Variability and Incident Disease in Older Women: The Iowa Women's Health Study," *International Journal of Obesity and Related Metabolic Disorders* 21 (1997): 217–223; Suoma Saarni et al., "Weight Cycling of Athletes and Subsequent Weight Gain in Middleage," *International Journal of Obesity* 30 (2006): 1639–1644.

p. 65   *"We simply do not know whether a person who loses 20 lb":* Jerome Kassirer and Marcia Angell, "Losing Weight: An Ill-Fated New Year's Resolution," *New England Journal of Medicine* 338 (1998): 52–54.

p. 66   *average American women and men are overweight on the BMI scale:* Cynthia Ogden et al., "Mean Body Weight, Height, and Body Mass Index, United States, 1960–2002," Centers for Disease Control and Prevention, National Center for Health Statistics, *Advance Data* 347 (2004), www.cdc.gov/nchs/data/ad/ad347.pdf.

p. 66   *two-thirds of American adults fall into the overweight or obese range:* Cynthia Ogden et al., "Prevalence of Overweight and Obesity in the United States, 1999–2004," *Journal of the American Medical Association* 295 (2006): 1549–1555.

p. 66   *(an apple shape) may be at greater risk:* See, for example, Shankuan Zhu et al., "Race-Ethnicity-Specific Waist Circumference Cutoffs for Identifying Cardiovascular Disease Risk Factors," *American Journal of Clinical Nutrition* 81 (2005): 409–415; Youfa Wang et al., "Comparison of Abdominal Adiposity and Overall Obesity in Predicting Type 2 Diabetes among Men," *American Journal of Clinical Nutrition* 81 (2005): 555–563; Tobias Pischon et al., "Body Size and Risk of Colon and Rectal Cancer in the European Prospective Investigation into Cancer and Nutrition (EPIC)," *Journal of the National Cancer Institute* 98 (2006): 920–931.

p. 66   *an implausibly high figure contradicted by CDC research:* Katherine Flegal et al., "Excess Deaths Associated with Underweight, Overweight, and Obesity," *Journal of the American Medical Association* 293 (2005): 1861–1867.

p. 67   *blame weight issues for everything from suicides to global warming:* Gina Kolata, "For a World of Woes, We Blame Cookie Monsters," *New York Times*, October 29, 2006.

p. 67   *"economically will make AIDS look like the common cold":* Suzanne Somers, *Today Show*, NBC News, transcript, January 6, 2003.

p. 67   *"we are facing a public health disaster":* Dr. Mark Hyman, audio message, www.ultrametabolism.com.

p. 67   *higher weight associated with greater risk of earlier death:* Kenneth Adams et al., "Overweight, Obesity, and Mortality in a Large Prospective Cohort of Persons 50 to 71 Years Old," *New England Journal of Medicine* 355 (2006): 763–778; Eugenia Calle et al., "Body-Mass Index and Mortality in a Prospective Cohort of U.S. Adults," *New England Journal of Medicine* 341 (1999): 1097–1105; JoAnn Manson et al., "Body Weight and Mortality among Women," *New England Journal of Medicine* 333 (1995): 677–685.

p. 67   *people who are overweight are not at increased risk:* Katherine Flegal et al., "Cause-Specific Excess Deaths Associated with Underweight, Overweight, and Obesity," *Journal of the American Medical Association* 298 (2007): 2028–

2037; Abel Romero-Corral et al., "Association of Bodyweight with Total Mortality and with Cardiovascular Events in Coronary Artery Disease: A Systematic Review of Cohort Studies," *Lancet* 368 (2006): 666–678; Richard Troiano et al., "The Relationship between Body Weight and Mortality: A Quantitative Analysis of Combined Information from Existing Studies," *International Journal of Obesity* 20 (1996): 63–75.

p. 68   *African Americans and older people may have higher ideal BMIs:* Ramon Durazo-Arvizu et al., "Mortality and Optimal Body Mass Index in a Sample of the U.S. Population," *American Journal of Epidemiology* 147 (1998): 739–749; María Corrada et al., "Association of Body Mass Index and Weight Change with All-Cause Mortality in the Elderly," *American Journal of Epidemiology* 163 (2006): 938–949.

p. 68   *adverse effects of obesity:* See, for example, Elisabeth Luder et al., "Body Mass Index and the Risk of Asthma in Adults," *Respiratory Medicine* 98 (2004): 29–37; Reiko Suzuki et al., "Body Weight and Postmenopausal Breast Cancer Risk Defined by Estrogen and Progesterone Receptor Status among Swedish Women: A Prospective Cohort Study," *International Journal of Cancer* 119 (2006): 1683–1689; Anna Peeters et al., "Adult Obesity and the Burden of Disability throughout Life," *Obesity Research* 12 (2004): 1145–1151.

p. 68   *nearly half of U.S. adult women and one-third of men trying to lose weight:* Edward Weiss et al., "Weight-Control Practices among U.S. Adults, 2001–2002," *American Journal of Preventive Medicine* 31 (2006): 18–24.

p. 68   *annual spending on weight loss products and services:* Ibid.

p. 68   *research suggests preventing weight gain is a good idea:* See, for example, Graham Colditz et al., "Weight Gain as a Risk Factor for Clinical Diabetes Mellitus in Women," *Annals of Internal Medicine* 122 (1995): 481–486; Rebecca Sedjo et al., "Change in Body Size and the Risk of Colorectal Adenomas," *Cancer Epidemiology, Biomarkers and Prevention* 16 (2007): 526–531.

p. 69   *"no exercise-needed approach to weight loss":* Advertisement for Arthur Agatston's book *The South Beach Diet, New York Times,* June 13, 2003. In the book, the author does recommend exercise but devotes only a few pages to the subject.

p. 69   *it's possible to be both fit and fat:* Chong Do Lee, Steven Blair, and Andrew Jackson, "Cardiorespiratory Fitness, Body Composition, and All-Cause and Cardiovascular Disease Mortality in Men," *American Journal of Clinical Nutrition* 69 (1999): 373–380.

p. 69   *fitness level is a more important contributor:* Timothy Wessel et al., "Relationship of Physical Fitness vs. Body Mass Index with Coronary Artery Disease and Cardiovascular Events in Women," *Journal of the American Medical Association* 292 (2004): 1179–1187.

p. 69   *some researchers don't agree that fitness trumps fatness:* Frank Hu et al., "Adiposity as Compared with Physical Activity in Predicting Mortality among Women," *New England Journal of Medicine* 2004 (351): 2694–2703.

p. 69   *"super-bodied athletes":* Laura Fraser, *Losing It: America's Obsession with Weight and the Industry That Feeds on It* (New York: Dutton, 1997), 270.

p. 70   *by opting for less energy-dense foods:* Jenny Ledikwe et al., "Dietary Energy Density Is Associated with Energy Intake and Weight Status in U.S. Adults," *American Journal of Clinical Nutrition* 83 (2006): 1362–1368; Julia Ello-Martin et al., "The Influence of Food Portion Size and Energy Density on Energy Intake: Implications for Weight Management," *American Journal of Clinical Nutrition* 82 (2005): 236S–241S.

p. 70   *oblivious to how much we're consuming:* Brian Wansink, Koert van Ittersum, and James Painter, "Ice Cream Illusions: Bowls, Spoons, and Self-Served Portion Sizes," *American Journal of Preventive Medicine* 31 (2006): 240–243; Brian Wansink, James Painter, and Jill North, "Bottomless Bowls: Why Visual Cues of Portion Sizes May Influence Intake," *Obesity Research* 13 (2005): 93–100.

p. 71   *a strategy called "Health at Every Size":* Linda Bacon et al., "Size Acceptance and Intuitive Eating Improve Health for Obese, Female Chronic Dieters," *Journal of the American Dietetic Association* 105 (2005): 929–936.

p. 72   *a* Consumer Reports *survey:* "The Truth about Dieting," *Consumer Reports,* June 2002, 26–31.

4. ADVERTISEMENTS

p. 76   *more than $23 billion a year:* National Institutes of Health, "State-of-the-Science Conference Statement: Multivitamin/Mineral Supplements and Chronic Disease Prevention," *Annals of Internal Medicine* 145 (2006): 364–71.

p. 76   *"are not allowed to make claims for their safety or effectiveness":* Harris Interactive, "Widespread Ignorance of Regulation and Labeling of Vitamins, Minerals, and Food Supplements," *Health Care News,* December 23, 2002, www .harrisinteractive.com/news/newsletters/healthnews/HI_HealthCareNews 2002Vol2_Iss23.pdf.

p. 77   *ephedra deaths and adverse events:* Paul Shekelle et al., "Efficacy and Safety of Ephedra and Ephedrine for Weight Loss and Athletic Performance: A Meta-analysis," *Journal of the American Medical Association* 289 (2003): 1537–1545.

p. 77   *"two quite questionable assumptions":* Marion Nestle, *What to Eat* (New York: North Point Press, 2006), 471.

p. 77   *"EPHEDRA IS BACK!":* Www.ephedraburn.com, accessed September 1, 2007. No longer available.

p. 78   *the agency has managed to crack down on only a handful:* For a description of these and other actions the FTC has taken, see www.ftc.gov.

p. 79   *"We obviously must make some difficult choices"*: Sheila F. Anthony, remarks
         before the Food and Drug Law Institute, 45th Annual Educational Con-
         ference, Washington, D.C., April 16, 2002.

p. 79   *lawsuits filed against ephedra supplement makers:* Ford Fessenden, "Studies of
         Dietary Supplements Come under Growing Scrutiny," *New York Times,*
         June 23, 2003.

p. 80   *this research involved not the supplements being advertised:* Edmund Chein,
         Daniel Vogt, and Cass Terry, "Clinical Experiences Using a Low-Dose,
         High-Frequency Human Growth Hormone Treatment Regimen," *Journal
         of Advancement in Medicine* 12 (1999): 183–191. Many of the ads erro-
         neously list Cass Terry as "L. Casserry."

p. 80   *A far more rigorous GH study:* Daniel Rudman et al., "Effects of Human
         Growth Hormone in Men over 60 Years Old," *New England Journal of*
         Medicine 323 (1990): 1–6.

p. 80   *"makes you look and feel 20 YEARS YOUNGER!":* See www.livelean02.com.

p. 80   *"they are being misled":* Jeffrey Drazen, "Inappropriate Advertising of Die-
         tary Supplements," *New England Journal of Medicine* 348 (2003): 777–778.

p. 81   *"The Science behind Hoodia Gordonii":* See www.hoodithin.com/about.php.

p. 82   *beta-carotene and lower rates of cancer and heart disease:* See, for example, Geert
         van Poppel and R. Alexandra Goldbohm, "Epidemiologic Evidence for
         Beta-Carotene and Cancer Prevention," *American Journal of Clinical Nutri-
         tion* 62 (1995): 1393S–1402S; Lenore Kohlmeier and Susan Hastings, "Epi-
         demiologic Evidence of a Role of Carotenoids in Cardiovascular Disease
         Prevention," *American Journal of Clinical Nutrition* 52 (1995): 1370S–1376S.

p. 83   *smokers who took beta-carotene supplements:* The Alpha-Tocopherol Beta
         Carotene Cancer Prevention Study Group, "The Effect of Vitamin E and
         Beta Carotene on the Incidence of Lung Cancer and Other Cancers in
         Male Smokers," *New England Journal of Medicine* 330 (1994): 1029–1035;
         Gilbert Omenn et al., "Effects of a Combination of Beta Carotene and
         Vitamin A on Lung Cancer and Cardiovascular Disease," *New England
         Journal of Medicine* 334 (1996): 1150–1155.

p. 83   *15 million listeners:* Alan Farnham, "After Paul Harvey, What?" Forbes.com,
         June 5, 2006, http://members.forbes.com/forbes/2006/0605/050.html.

p. 83   *"He has a way of taking the essence of any product":* Ibid. The quote is from
         Neill Walsdorf Jr. of Mission Pharmacal, which sold the Citracal brand to
         Bayer Health Care in 2007.

p. 83   *Citracal radio ads:* Accessed through www.citracal.com, June 1, 2007; ads are
         no longer on the site.

p. 84   *calcium's effect on cholesterol levels:* Ian Reid et al., "Effects of Calcium Supple-
         mentation on Serum Lipid Concentrations in Normal Older Women: A
         Randomized Controlled Trial," *American Journal of Medicine* 112 (2002):
         343–347. But this study found no effect: Roberd Bostick et al., "Effect of

Calcium Supplementation on Serum Cholesterol and Blood Pressure,"
Archives of Family Medicine 9 (2000): 31–39.

p. 84   *Citracal and greater increases in bone density:* Ian Reid et al., "Randomized
Controlled Trial of Calcium in Healthy Older Women," *American Journal
of Medicine* 119 (2006): 777–785.

p. 84   *Various efforts to pool data from multiple studies:* Beverley Shea et al., "Meta-
Analysis of Calcium Supplementation for the Prevention of Postmenopausal
Osteoporosis," *Endocrine Reviews* 23 (2002): 552–559; Alison Avenell et al.,
"Vitamin D and Vitamin D Analogues for Preventing Fractures Associated
with Involutional and Post-Menopausal Osteoporosis," *Cochrane Database of
Systematic Reviews* 4 (1996), updated April 2005, www.cochrane.org/reviews/
en/ab000227.html; Benjamin Tang et al., "Use of Calcium or Calcium in
Combination with Vitamin D Supplementation to Prevent Fractures and
Bone Loss in People Aged 50 Years and Older: A Meta-Analysis," *Lancet* 370
(2007): 657–666.

p. 84   *Women's Health Initiative calcium trial:* Rebecca Jackson et al., "Calcium plus
Vitamin D Supplementation and the Risk of Fractures," *New England
Journal of Medicine* 354 (2006): 669–683.

p. 84   *"any benefit of calcium plus vitamin D":* Joel Finkelstein, "Calcium plus Vitamin D for Postmenopausal Women—Bone Appétit?" *New England Journal
of Medicine* 354 (2006): 750–752.

p. 85   *Research involving Finnish smokers:* Olli Heinonen et al., "Prostate Cancer
and Supplementation with Alpha-Tocopherol and Beta-Carotene: Incidence and Mortality in a Controlled Trial," *Journal of the National Cancer
Institute* 90 (1998): 440–446.

p. 87   *A panel of experts convened by the National Institutes of Health:* National
Institutes of Health, "State-of-the-Science Conference Statement."

p. 87   *folic acid and neural-tube birth defects:* Andrew Czeizel and Istvan Dudas,
"Prevention of the First Occurrence of Neural-Tube Defects by Peri-
conceptional Vitamin Supplementation," *New England Journal of Medicine*
327 (1992): 1832–1835.

p. 87   *"a personalized protocol of specially formulated nutraceuticals":* See www.suracell
.com/faqs/index.aspx#7.

p. 87   *GAO investigation of genetic tests:* U.S. Government Accountability Office,
"Nutrigenetic Testing: Tests Purchased from Four Web Sites Mislead
Consumers," statement of Gregory Kutz, testimony before the Special
Committee on Aging, U.S. Senate, July 27, 2006, www.gao.gov/new.items/
d06977t.pdf.

p. 89   *an investigation by the Center for Science in the Public Interest:* David Schardt,
"Supplementing Their Income: How Celebrities Turn Trust into Cash,"
Nutrition Action Healthletter, January/February 2006, www.cspinet.org/nah/
01_06/sup_can.pdf.

p. 89   "caveat emptor — *buyer beware!*": Andrew Weil, *Healthy Aging: A Lifelong
        Guide to Your Physical and Spiritual Well-Being* (New York: Knopf, 2005),
        176.

5. GOVERNMENT CAMPAIGNS

p. 94   *half of those who suffer heart attacks:* Paul Ridker et al., "C-Reactive Protein
        and Other Markers of Inflammation in the Prediction of Cardiovascular
        Disease in Women," *New England Journal of Medicine* 342 (2000): 836–843.

p. 94   *"well-earned reputation as the heart's primary nemesis":* Alice Park, "Beyond
        Cholesterol," *Time,* November 25, 2002, 74.

p. 95   *NCEP mission:* National Cholesterol Education Program, "Program
        Description," www.nhlbi.nih.gov/about/ncep.

p. 95   *25 percent of American adults had high cholesterol:* Christopher Semposet
        et al., "Prevalence of High Cholesterol among US Adults: An Update
        Based on Guidelines from the Second Report of the National Cholesterol
        Education Program Adult Treatment Panel," *Journal of the American
        Medical Association* 269 (1993): 3009–3014.

p. 95   *"It's a mammoth intervention":* Dr. James Cleeman quoted in Thomas
        Moore, *Heart Failure: A Critical Inquiry into American Medicine and the
        Revolution in Heart Care* (New York: Random House, 1989), 65.

p. 95   *typical print message:* The two print ads can be found in National Heart,
        Lung, and Blood Institute, "A Communications Strategy for Public
        Education: The National Cholesterol Program," NIH Publication no. 94-
        3292, November 1994.

p. 96   *93 percent . . . had heard of high cholesterol:* Beth Schucker et al., "Change in
        Cholesterol Awareness and Action: Results from National Physician and
        Public Surveys," *Archives of Internal Medicine* 151 (1991): 666–673.

p. 96   *2001 survey:* Ira Nash et al., "Contemporary Awareness and Understanding
        of Cholesterol as a Risk Factor: Results of an American Heart Association
        National Survey," *Archives of Internal Medicine* 163 (2003): 1597–1600.

p. 96   *proportion of people getting tested:* Susan Schober et al., "High Serum Total
        Cholesterol—An Indicator for Monitoring Cholesterol Lowering Efforts:
        U.S. Adults, 2005–2006," NCHS Data Brief No. 2, National Center for
        Health Statistics, December 2007, www.cdc.gov/nchs/data/databriefs/db02
        .pdf. For 1986 statistics, see Schucker et al., "Change in Cholesterol Aware-
        ness and Action."

p. 96   *average cholesterol levels have declined:* Schober, "High Serum Total Choles-
        terol"; Margaret Carroll et al., "Trends in Serum Lipids and Lipoproteins
        of Adults, 1960–2002," *Journal of the American Medical Association* 294
        (2005): 1773–1781.

p. 97   *messages based "firmly on sound scientific evidence":* National Cholesterol Edu-
        cation Program, "Program Description."

p. 97   *Framingham findings:* William Kannel et al., "Serum Cholesterol, Lipo-proteins, and the Risk of Coronary Heart Disease: The Framingham Study," *Annals of Internal Medicine* 74 (1971): 1–12.

p. 97   *As subjects got older, the risk . . . appeared to decline:* Richard Kronmal et al., "Total Serum Cholesterol Levels and Mortality Risk as a Function of Age: A Report Based on the Framingham Data," *Archives of Internal Medicine* 153 (1993): 1065–1073.

p. 97   *also cast doubt on the dangers of high cholesterol in the elderly:* Bruce Psaty et al., "The Association between Lipid Levels and the Risks of Incident Myo-cardial Infarction, Stroke, and Total Mortality: The Cardiovascular Health Study," *Journal of the American Geriatrics Society* 52 (2004): 1639–1647; Harlan Krumholz et al., "Lack of Association between Cholesterol and Coronary Heart Disease Mortality and Morbidity and All-Cause Mortality in Persons Older than 70 Years," *Journal of the American Medical Association* 272 (1994): 1335–1340; Irwin Schatz et al., "Cholesterol and All-Cause Mortality in Elderly People from the Honolulu Heart Program: A Cohort Study," *Lancet* 358 (2001): 351–355; Nicole Schupf et al., "Relationship between Plasma Lipids and All-Cause Mortality in Nondemented Elderly," *Journal of the American Geriatrics Society* 53 (2005): 219–226.

p. 97   *"cholesterol lowering is important for young, middle-aged, and older adults":* National Cholesterol Education Program, "Live Healthier, Live Longer," www.nhlbisupport.com/chd1/did.htm.

p. 98   *people over 65 can "benefit greatly":* Ibid., www.nhlbisupport.com/chd1/faq1 .htm.

p. 98   *a survey of healthy people age 65 and older:* Esprin Reddy, Nan Kreher, and John Hickner, "How Concerned Are Elderly Patients without Coronary Heart Disease about Hypercholesterolemia and Heart Disease? An UPRNet Study," *Journal of Family Practice* 46 (1998): 227–232.

p. 98   *"What you eat greatly affects your blood cholesterol levels":* National Heart, Lung, and Blood Institute, "Your Guide to Lowering Your Cholesterol with TLC," NIH Publication no. 06-5235, December 2005, 19.

p. 99   *risk factors for heart disease:* National Cholesterol Education Program, "Live Healthier, Live Longer," www.nhlbisupport.com/chd1/chdexp1.htm.

p. 99   *cholesterol level "has a lot to do with your chances of getting heart disease":* National Cholesterol Education Program, "High Blood Cholesterol: What You Need to Know," NIH Publication no. 05-3290, June 2005.

p. 99   *Framingham Risk Assessment Tool:* Examples are from the risk calculator avail-able at http://hp2010.nhlbihin.net/atpiii/calculator.asp. Though this tool can provide a rough estimate of risk, it has been criticized for taking too few factors into account. A more complete tool can be found on the Ameri-can Heart Association's Web site at www.americanheart.org/presenter.jhtml ?identifier=3003499#what.

p. 99   *"your LDL level is a good indicator of your risk":* National Cholesterol Education Program, "Live Healthier, Live Longer," www.nhlbisupport.com/chd1/treatment.htm.

p. 99   *high cholesterol is a "serious condition":* National Heart, Lung, and Blood Institute, "Your Guide to Lowering Your Cholesterol with TLC," 1.

p. 100 *three consequences of labeling risk factors as diseases:* Lynn Payer, *Disease-Mongers: How Doctors, Drug Companies, and Insurers Are Making You Feel Sick* (New York: Wiley, 1992), 172–173. For more on disease-mongering, see Ray Moynihan and David Henry, "The Fight against Disease Mongering: Generating Knowledge for Action," *PLoS Medicine* 3 (2006): e191, http://medicine.plosjournals.org/perlserv/?request=get-document&doi=10.1371/journal.pmed.0030191&ct=1.

p. 101 *a 2004 NCEP panel called for even more aggressive use:* Scott Grundy et al., "Implications of Recent Clinical Trials for the National Cholesterol Education Program Adult Treatment Panel III Guidelines," *Circulation* 110 (2004): 227–239.

p. 101 *More than thirty physicians and research scientists:* John Abramson et al., "Petition to the National Institutes of Health Seeking an Independent Review Panel to Re-evaluate the National Cholesterol Education Program Guidelines," September 23, 2004, www.cspinet.org/integrity/press/200409231.html.

p. 101 *Eight of the nine experts:* For a list of panelists and their financial disclosures, see National Cholesterol Education Program, "ATP III Update 2004: Financial Disclosures," www.nhlbi.nih.gov/guidelines/cholesterol/atp3upd04_disclose.htm.

p. 101 *panelists are chosen for their "scientific and medical expertise":* Letter from Barbara Alving, acting director of NHLBI, to Merrill Goozner, October 22, 2004, www.nhlbi.nih.gov/guidelines/cholesterol/response.pdf.

p. 101 *"when companies with identical interests":* Jerome Kassirer, "Why Should We Swallow What These Studies Say?" *Washington Post*, April 1, 2004.

p. 102 *secondary prevention studies:* See, for example, Scandinavian Simvastatin Survival Study Group, "Randomised Trial of Cholesterol Lowering in 4,444 Patients with Coronary Heart Disease: The Scandinavian Simvastatin Survival Study (4S)," *Lancet* 344 (1994): 1383–1389; Long-Term Intervention with Pravastatin in Ischaemic Disease (LIPID) Study Group, "Prevention of Cardiovascular Events and Death with Pravastatin in Patients with Coronary Heart Disease and a Broad Range of Initial Cholesterol Levels," *New England Journal of Medicine* 339 (1998): 1349–1357; Heart Protection Study Collaborative Group, "MRC/BHF Heart Protection Study of Cholesterol Lowering with Simvastatin in 20,538 High-Risk Individuals: A Randomised Placebo-Controlled Trial," *Lancet* 360 (2002): 7–22.

p. 102   *value . . . isn't as clear-cut when it comes to primary prevention:* Paaladinesh Thavendiranathan et al., "Primary Prevention of Cardiovascular Diseases with Statin Therapy," *Archives of Internal Medicine* 166 (2006): 2307–2313.

p. 102   *as many as 75 percent of people on statins:* Isabelle Savoie and Arminée Kazanjian, "Utilization of Lipid-Lowering Drugs in Men and Women: A Reflection of the Research Evidence?" *Journal of Clinical Epidemiology* 55 (2002): 95–101.

p. 102   *Abramson and Wright analysis:* John Abramson and James Wright, "Are Lipid-Lowering Guidelines Evidence-Based?" *Lancet* 369 (2007): 168–169.

p. 102   *"You're expecting me to take a pill":* James Wright quoted in Shelley Wood, "*Lancet* Comment Questions Benefit of Statins in Primary Prevention," *Heartwire,* January 25, 2007, www.medscape.com/viewarticle/551324.

p. 102   *Women without heart disease didn't seem to be helped:* See Judith Walsh and Michael Pignone, "Drug Treatment of Hyperlipidemia in Women," *Journal of the American Medical Association* 291 (2004): 2243–2252.

p. 102   *"Such a sweeping recommendation":* John Abramson, *Overdosed America: The Broken Promise of American Medicine* (New York: HarperCollins, 2004), 140.

p. 103   *the number of older people on statins has grown substantially:* Carroll et al., "Trends in Serum Lipids and Lipoproteins."

p. 103   *perhaps exceeding $100 billion:* Thavendiranathan et al., "Primary Prevention of Cardiovascular Diseases with Statin Therapy."

p. 103   *People who are over 80 (especially women):* For an overview of statin risks in the elderly, see Beatrice Golomb, "Statin Adverse Effects: Implications for the Elderly," *Geriatric Times* 5 (2004): 18–20.

p. 104   *impaired memory and thinking:* Ibid.

p. 104   *A trial involving people age 70 and older:* James Shepherd et al., "Pravastatin in Elderly Individuals at Risk of Vascular Disease (PROSPER): A Randomised Controlled Trial," *Lancet* 360 (2002): 1623–1630.

p. 104   *Several other efforts to pool results from multiple studies:* Krista Dale et al., "Statins and Cancer Risk: A Meta-Analysis," *Journal of the American Medical Association* 295 (2006): 74–80; Colin Baigent et al., "Efficacy and Safety of Cholesterol-Lowering Treatment: Prospective Meta-Analysis of Data from 90,056 Participants in 14 Randomised Trials of Statins," *Lancet* 366 (2005): 1267–1278.

p. 104   *"disturbing" finding about statins and cancer:* Alawi Alsheikh-Ali et al., "Effect of the Magnitude of Lipid Lowering on Risk of Elevated Liver Enzymes, Rhabdomyolysis, and Cancer: Insights from Large Randomized Statin Trials," *Journal of the American College of Cardiology* 50 (2007): 409–418.

p. 104   *epidemiological studies that have linked low cholesterol to cancer:* See, for example, David Jacobs et al., "Report of the Conference on Low Blood Cholesterol: Mortality Associations," *Circulation* 86 (1992): 1046–1060; Carlos

Iribarren et al., "Low Serum Cholesterol and Mortality: Which Is the Cause and Which Is the Effect?" *Circulation* 92 (1995): 2396–2403.

p. 105 *"Most heart disease results from the way we live":* John Abramson and Merrill Goozner, "Pills to Avoid Heart Attacks? Hard to Swallow," *Los Angeles Times,* October 21, 2005.

p. 106 *"has transformed what would otherwise":* James Cleeman and Claude Lenfant, "The National Cholesterol Education Program: Progress and Prospects," *Journal of the American Medical Association* 280 (1998): 2099–2104.

p. 106 *Cholesterol Low Down:* See www.cholesterollowdown.org.

p. 106 *"the messages of cholesterol education":* Cleeman and Lenfant, "The National Cholesterol Education Program."

6. CELEBRITIES

p. 109 *Oprah calls full-body scans "miraculous": The Oprah Winfrey Show,* transcript, October 2, 2000.

p. 110 *Oprah's on-air test did for full-body scans:* Liz Kowalczyk, "Full-Body Disagreement: Harvard Doctors Offer Scans That Many in Medical Establishment Spurn," *Boston Globe,* June 28, 2002.

p. 110 *the dose of radiation they deliver can be high:* Center for Devices and Radiological Health, U.S. Food and Drug Administration, "Whole-Body CT Screening—Should I or Shouldn't I Get One?" www.fda.gov/cdrh/ct/ screening.html.

p. 110 *In one survey, nearly 87 percent of adults:* Lisa Schwartz et al., "Enthusiasm for Cancer Screening in the United States," *Journal of the American Medical Association* 291 (2004): 71–78.

p. 111 *"Katie Couric Effect":* Peter Cram et al., "The Impact of a Celebrity Promotional Campaign on the Use of Colon Cancer Screening," *Archives of Internal Medicine* 163 (2003): 1601–1605.

p. 111 *second leading cause of cancer deaths:* American Cancer Society, "Cancer Facts and Figures 2007," www.cancer.org/downloads/STT/CAFF2007PW Secured.pdf.

p. 111 *USPSTF colon cancer screening recommendations:* U.S. Preventive Services Task Force, "Screening for Colorectal Cancer," July 2002, www.ahrq.gov/ clinic/uspstf/uspscolo.htm#summary. For more on USPSTF, see www.ahrq .gov/clinic/uspstfab.htm.

p. 111 *They all recommend one of several options:* Sidney Winawer et al., "Colorectal Cancer Screening and Surveillance: Clinical Guidelines and Rationale— Update Based on New Evidence," *Gastroenterology* 124 (2003): 544–560; American Cancer Society, "Can Colorectal Polyps and Cancer Be Found Early? Colorectal Cancer Screening," www.cancer.org/docroot/CRI/ content/ CRI_2_4_3X_Can_colon_and_rectum_cancer_be_found_early.asp.

p. 112   *to detect one cancer among people in their 40s:* Thomas Imperiale et al., "Results of Screening Colonoscopy among Persons 40 to 49 Years of Age," *New England Journal of Medicine* 346 (2002): 1781–1785.

p. 112   *"All the doctors I know":* Joanna Powell, "Katie Couric's Story: Life after Loss," *Good Housekeeping,* October 1998.

p. 112   *"She used her position":* Gary Schwitzer, "One Complication of the Couric Crusade," www.tc.umn.edu/%7Eschwitz/Couriccampaign.htm.

p. 112   *average age of* Today Show *viewers:* Cram et al., "Impact of a Celebrity Promotional Campaign."

p. 112   *Almost half of people 50 and older don't get screened:* Centers for Disease Control and Prevention, "Increased Use of Colorectal Cancer Tests—United States, 2002 and 2004," *Morbidity and Mortality Weekly Report* 55 (2006): 308–311.

p. 113   *the most frequently diagnosed cancer in men:* American Cancer Society, "Cancer Facts and Figures 2007."

p. 113   *only about 25 to 30 percent of those who are biopsied:* National Cancer Institute, Fact Sheet, "The Prostate-Specific Antigen Test (PSA): Questions and Answers," www.cancer.gov/cancertopics/factsheet/Detection/PSA.

p. 114   *USPSTF prostate cancer screening recommendations:* U.S. Preventive Services Task Force, "Screening for Prostate Cancer," December 2002, www.ahrq.gov/clinic/uspstf/uspsprca.htm.

p. 114   *the CDC urges each man to discuss:* Centers for Disease Control and Prevention, "Prostate Cancer Screening: A Decision Guide," www.cdc.gov/cancer/prostate/publications/decisionguide.

p. 114   *Prostate Cancer Foundation recommendation:* Prostate Cancer Foundation, "Detection and Screening," www.prostatecancerfoundation.org/site/c.itIWK2OSG/b.47285/k.CCF1/Detection__Screening.htm.

p. 114   *"Believe me, early detection is the key":* See the video message on Palmer's Web site at www.arniesarmybattles.com/watch_video.html.

p. 114   *"I know that there are also a lot of men":* Arnold Palmer quoted in Barbara Payne, "The Legend Continues . . . after Prostate Cancer," interview with PROACT, www.yourfamilyshealth.com/cancer/prostate/arnold_palmer/.

p. 114   *"If you're over 50 or in a high risk group":* Mike Falcon, "Giuliani Defeats Prostate Cancer," Spotlight Health, October 14, 2002, www.usatoday.com/news/health/spotlighthealth/2002-10-14-giuliani_x.htm.

p. 115   *they get tested at least* twice *a year:* John Morgan, "Baseball Stars 'Double Up' Prostate Cancer," Spotlight Health, July 18, 2003, www.usatoday.com/news/health/spotlighthealth/2003-07-18-baseball_x.htm; Gary Gately, "Pro Baseball Goes to Bat against Prostate Cancer," *HealthDay,* July 16, 2003.

p. 115   *five-year survival rates for prostate cancer:* American Cancer Society,

"Overview: Prostate Cancer—Prostate Cancer Survival Rates," June 2007, www.cancer.org/docroot/CRI/content/CRI_2_2_6x_Prostate_Cancer _Survival_Rates.asp?sitearea=.

p. 115 *"another excuse":* The letter, dated March 13, 2002, is posted online at www .usrf.org/breakingnews/bn_020319_Time_PSA_testing/bn_020319_NPCC _letter.html. The article that prompted Atkins's letter was Christine Gorman, "What's a Guy to Do?" *Time,* March 18, 2002, 98.

p. 115 *seen or heard celebrities talking about PSA testing:* Robin Larson et al., "Celebrity Endorsements of Cancer Screening," *Journal of the National Cancer Institute* 97 (2005): 693–695.

p. 116 *"The reason to get tested for cancer":* H. Gilbert Welch, *Should I Be Tested for Cancer? Maybe Not and Here's Why* (Berkeley: University of California Press, 2004), 188.

p. 117 *fall into this gray zone of osteopenia:* Centers for Disease Control and Prevention, National Health and Nutrition Examination Survey, "Osteoporosis," www.cdc.gov/nchs/data/nhanes/databriefs/osteoporosis.pdf.

p. 117 *disease-mongering:* Ray Moynihan, Iona Heath, and David Henry, "Selling Sickness: The Pharmaceutical Industry and Disease Mongering," *British Medical Journal* 324 (2002): 886–891.

p. 117 *medication for osteopenia:* Sundeep Khosla and Joseph Melton, "Osteopenia," *New England Journal of Medicine* 356 (2007): 2293–2300.

p. 117 *A panel of experts convened by the National Institutes of Health:* "Osteoporosis Prevention, Diagnosis, and Therapy," NIH Consensus Development Conference Statement, March 27–29, 2000, http://consensus.nih.gov/2000/ 2000Osteoporosis111html.htm.

p. 117 *USPSTF osteoporosis screening recommendation:* U.S. Preventive Services Task Force, "Screening for Osteoporosis in Postmenopausal Women," September 2002, www.ahrq.gov/clinic/3rduspstf/osteoporosis/osteorr .htm.

p. 117 *"bone density tests are the most important thing":* "The Importance of Osteoporosis Testing," www.drdonnica.com/display.asp?article=1173.

p. 118 *"absolutely criminal":* Tammy Collins Carter, "Rita Moreno Takes AARP Stage to Confront Osteoporosis," *Orlando Sentinel,* May 18, 2000.

p. 118 *Debbie Reynolds's letter to Ann Landers: Washington Post,* January 21, 2000.

p. 118 *"If you test for it early enough":* Joan Tarshis, "Celebrities Reveal Their Secrets," *Parade,* March 19, 2000, 10–12.

p. 118 *"Tell them you really want to know your T-score":* John Morgan, "Meredith Vieira Takes Keen View on Osteoporosis," Spotlight Health, June 6, 2003, www.usatoday.com/news/health/spotlighthealth/2003-06-06-Vieira_x .htm.

p. 118   *"I was surprised when I learned":* "Meredith Vieira Shares Her 'View' about 'Being Beautiful to the Bone,'" PR Newswire, May 5, 2003.

p. 118   *Merck has made screening a centerpiece of its marketing efforts:* For more, see Susan Kelleher, "Disease Expands through Marriage of Marketing and Machines," *Seattle Times,* June 28, 2005.

p. 119   *Vieira's appearance on* Good Morning America: *Good Morning America,* ABC News, transcript, May 27, 2003.

p. 119   *In 2002, Salon.com and the* New York Times *revealed:* Lawrence Goodman, "Celebrity Pill Pushers," Salon.com, July 11, 2002, http://dir.salon.com/ story/mwt/feature/2002/07/11/celebrity_drugs/index1.html; Melody Petersen, "Heartfelt Advice, Hefty Fees," *New York Times,* August 11, 2002.

p. 119   *"still love celebrity health campaigns":* Bob Brody, "Celebrity Health Campaigns: The Next Generation," www.ogilvypr.com/expert-views/ celebrity-health-campaigns.cfm.

p. 121   *USPSTF cardiac CT screening recommendations:* U.S. Preventive Services Task Force, "Screening for Coronary Heart Disease," February 2004, www .ahrq.gov/clinic/uspstf/uspsacad.htm.

p. 121   *the test may be useful for certain people:* Matthew Budoff et al., "Assessment of Coronary Artery Disease by Cardiac Computed Tomography," *Circulation* 114 (2006): 1761–1791.

p. 121   *"Could these deaths have been prevented?":* Advanced Body Scan of Newport, www.newportbodyscan.com/Preventable_Deaths.htm.

p. 121   *"limitations of stress tests":* Colorado Heart and Body Imaging (Denver), "Clinton Heart Disease Reveals Misconceptions about Testing," press release, September 29, 2004. The physician quoted is Harvey Hecht, MD.

p. 122   *"saved Mr. Clinton from a trip to the operating room":* Colorado Heart and Body Imaging (Denver), ad supplied June 13, 2006, by Dr. James Ehrlich, medical director and founder of the clinic.

p. 122   *"Don't be as dumb":* Ohio Heart, Columbus, Ohio. Ad supplied July 5, 2006, by Bruce Friedman, president of Heart Check America. For more on this and other ads mentioning Bill Clinton, see Eric Barnes, "Scan Centers Take Heart in 'Clinton Syndrome,'" September 16, 2004, www .auntminnie.com.

p. 122   *Though some research suggests otherwise:* Patrick O'Malley, Irwin Feuerstein, and Allen Taylor, "Impact of Electron Beam Tomography, with or without Case Management, on Motivation, Behavioral Change, and Cardiovascular Risk Profile," *Journal of the American Medical Association* 289 (2003): 2215– 2223.

p. 123   *Oprah was at it again: The Oprah Winfrey Show,* transcript, October 19, 2005.

7. HEALTH GROUPS

p. 127   *"We all need sunscreen"*: See www.playsafeinthesun.org/events/color_contest
_winners.html.

p. 128   *respondents were far more likely to list "apply sunscreen"*: Survey of 1,011 adults
age 18 and older, conducted by International Communications Research
(ICR) for Transitions Optical, March 9–13, 2006.

p. 128   *"Wear sunscreen. If I could offer you only one tip"*: Mary Schmich, "Advice,
Like Youth, Probably Just Wasted on the Young," *Chicago Tribune*, June 1,
1997.

p. 128   *we tend to stay in the sun longer:* Philippe Autier, Mathieu Boniol, and Jean-
François Doré, "Sunscreen Use and Increased Duration of Intentional Sun
Exposure: Still a Burning Issue," *International Journal of Cancer* 121 (2007):
1–5.

p. 129   *sunscreen sales have soared:* Information Resources Inc., cited in Lindsay
Elkins, "Here Comes the Sun," *Household and Personal Products Industry*
(Happi), March 1, 2007, www.happi.com/articles/2007/03/here-comes-the-
sun.php.

p. 129   *squamous cell carcinoma and use of sunscreen:* Richard Gallagher, "Sunscreens
in Melanoma and Skin Cancer Prevention," *Canadian Medical Association
Journal* 173 (2005): 244–245; Adele Green et al., "Daily Sunscreen Appli-
cation and Betacarotene Supplementation in Prevention of Basal-Cell and
Squamous-Cell Carcinomas of the Skin: A Randomised Controlled Trial,"
Lancet 354 (1999): 723–729.

p. 129   *basal and squamous cell cancers affect more than 1 million:* American Cancer
Society, "Skin Cancer Facts," www.cancer.org/docroot/PED/content/ped_7
_1_What_You_Need_To_Know_About_Skin_Cancer.asp?sitearea=&level.

p. 129   *roughly 8,000 Americans die of melanoma:* American Cancer Society, "Cancer
Facts and Figures 2007," www.cancer.org/downloads/STT/CAFF2007
PWSecured.pdf.

p. 129   *the rate of new cases is about six times higher:* H. Gilbert Welch, Steven Woloshin, and Lisa Schwartz, "Skin Biopsy Rates and Incidence of Melanoma:
Population Based Ecological Study," *British Medical Journal* 331 (2005): 481.

p. 130   *greater vigilance by doctors:* Ibid.

p. 130   *Two analyses that pooled results:* Leslie Dennis, Laura Beane Freeman, and
Marta Van Beek, "Sunscreen Use and the Risk for Melanoma: A Quanti-
tative Review," *Annals of Internal Medicine* 139 (2003): 966–978; Michael
Huncharek and Bruce Kupelnick, "Use of Topical Sunscreens and the Risk
of Malignant Melanoma: A Meta-Analysis of 9,067 Patients from 11 Case-
Control Studies," *American Journal of Public Health* 92 (2002): 1173–1177.

p. 130   *"no evidence of protective value":* Gallagher, "Sunscreens."

p. 130   *"sunscreens would have failed the tests"*: Olaf Gefeller of the University of
          Erlangen-Nuremberg in Germany, quoted by Damaris Christensen in
          "Data Still Cloudy on Association between Sunscreen Use and Melanoma
          Risk," *Journal of the National Cancer Institute* 95 (2003): 932–933.

p. 130   *when sunscreen-covered mice are exposed to UV light:* Peter Wolf, Cherrie
          Donawho, and Margaret Kripke, "Effect of Sunscreens on UV Radiation–
          Induced Enhancement of Melanoma Growth in Mice," *Journal of the
          National Cancer Institute* 86 (1994): 99–105.

p. 131   *newer formulations of sunscreen:* See, for example, Brian Diffey, "Sunscreens
          and Melanoma: The Future Looks Bright," *British Journal of Dermatology*
          153 (2005): 378–381.

p. 131   *UVA rays . . . may be an important contributor to melanoma:* S. Q. Wang et al.,
          "Ultraviolet A and Melanoma: A Review," *Journal of the American Academy
          of Dermatology* 44 (2001): 837–846.

p. 131   *the role of sun exposure in melanoma:* Jason Rivers, "Is There More than One
          Road to Melanoma?" *Lancet* 363 (2004): 728–730.

p. 131   *cover up or go indoors:* See Stephan Lautenschlager, Hans Christian Wulf,
          and Mark R. Pittelkow, "Photoprotection," *Lancet* 370 (2007): 528–537.

p. 132   *"sustaining support"*: Skin Cancer Foundation, "Corporate Council," www
          .skincancer.org/content/view/131/62/.

p. 132   *SCF lists these recommendations:* See www.skincancer.org/prevention/year-
          round-sun-protection.html.

p. 133   *products that claim to provide "broad-spectrum" protection:* "Sunscreens: Some
          Are Short on Protection," *Consumer Reports,* July 2007, 6; Helena Gonzalez
          et al., "Photostability of Commercial Sunscreens upon Sun Exposure
          and Irradiation by Ultraviolet Lamps," *BMC Dermatology* 7 (2007), www
          .biomedcentral.com/1471-5945/7/1. See also the Environmental Working
          Group's analysis of more than 900 sunscreens, available at www.cosmetics
          database.com/special/sunscreens/summary.php.

p. 133   *new rules were proposed in August 2007:* See "FDA Proposes New Rule for
          Sunscreen Products," www.fda.gov/bbs/topics/NEWS/2007/NEW01687
          .html.

p. 133   *the SCF seal has so far done nothing to fill the void:* In its response to the pro-
          posed FDA rule changes regarding sunscreen labeling, SCF says its seal of
          recommendation will incorporate the new FDA requirements. See www
          .skincancer.org/content/view/269/0/.

p. 134   *"cause marketing" relationship:* Len Lichtenfeld, "Skin Cancer and the *New
          York Times*," Dr. Len's Cancer Blog, July 11, 2007, ww.cancer.org/aspx/
          blog/Comments.aspx?id=158.

p. 134   *"there is no conflict of interest"*: Ibid.

p. 134   *"reduce the incidence of skin cancer by motivating people"*: Sun Safety Alliance, "Our Mission," www.sunsafetyalliance.org/wmspage.cfm?parm1=55.

p. 135   *"To stem this epidemic"*: Sun Safety Alliance, "Americans Get Failing Grade in Practicing Sun Safety beyond Beach or Pool," press release, June 21, 2004, www.sunsafetyalliance.org/user-assets/documents/SSA_pressrelease _6-04.pdf.

p. 135   *"long recognized as the first line of defense"*: Sun Safety Alliance, "RAFT Study and Sunscreen Usage," press release, October 9, 2003. The study to which Schneider referred was Rachel Haywood et al., "Sunscreens Inadequately Protect against Ultraviolet-A-Induced Free Radicals in Skin: Implications for Skin Aging and Melanoma," *Investigative Dermatology* 121 (2003): 862– 868.

p. 135   *"the alliance will expand the base of future customers"*: Molly Prior, "NACDS Sun Safety Alliance Rallies Industry in Fight against Skin Cancer," *Drug Store News*, June 17, 2002, http://findarticles.com/p/articles/mi_m3374/is_8 _24/ai_87511094.

p. 135   *"to focus people's attention on the simple actions"*: Sun Safety Alliance, "Sunscreen Use Down as Skin Cancer Rates Increase," press release, June 6, 2005, www.sunsafetyalliance.org/user-assets/Documents/060605 _SSA_Release .pdf.

p. 135   *persuaded Congress to pass a resolution:* HR 169, 109th Cong., June 7, 2005, www.govtrack.us/congress/bill.xpd?tab=summary&bill=hr109-169; S 167, 109th Cong., June 9, 2005, www.govtrack.us/congress/billtext.xpd?bill =sr109-167.

p. 136   *"primary protector against skin cancer"*: Sun Safety Alliance, "Sunscreen Use Down as Skin Cancer Rates Increase."

p. 136   *instructed to visit Coppertone's Web site:* See www.sunsafetyalliance.org/ user-assets/Documents/TeachingGuide.pdf.

p. 136   *"Get Sun-Certified Quiz"*: Ibid.

p. 136   *"install a pump full of sunscreen"*: "Sun Safety Alliance Announces Winners of Grant Competition and Letter-Writing Contest to President Bush," PR Newswire, June 12, 2003.

p. 136   *"commitment to building a national grassroots movement"*: Statement by Barbara Bush, June 2005, www.sunsafetyalliance.org/user-assets/Documents/ 060605_BB_Statement_LTR.pdf.

p. 137   *announcing the group's launch: Today Show,* NBC News, transcript, April 22, 2003.

p. 137   *a finding repeatedly cited by SSA:* Robert Stern, Milton Weinstein, and Stuart Baker, "Risk Reduction for Nonmelanoma Skin Cancer with Childhood Sunscreen Use," *Archives of Dermatology* 122 (1986): 537–545.

p. 138   *"self-serving advocacy group"*: Wolff System Technology, "American Academy of Dermatology Teams Up with Drug Stores and Coppertone to Mislead Sun-Tanners about Health Benefits of Sunshine," news release, April 16, 2004, www.wolffsystem.com/dermatology.html.

p. 138   *indoor tanning linked to a higher risk of melanoma*: International Agency for Research on Cancer Working Group on Artificial Ultraviolet Light and Skin Cancer, "The Association of Use of Sunbeds with Cutaneous Malignant Melanoma and Other Skin Cancers: A Systematic Review," *International Journal of Cancer* 120 (2007): 1116–1122.

p. 138   *sun exposure and lower incidence of cancers*: H. J. van der Rhee, E. de Vries, and J. W. Coebergh, "Does Sunlight Prevent Cancer? A Systematic Review," *European Journal of Cancer* 42 (2006): 2222–2232.

p. 138   *sun exposure and multiple sclerosis*: See, for example, Ingrid van der Mei et al., "Past Exposure to Sun, Skin Phenotype, and Risk of Multiple Sclerosis: Case Control Study," *British Medical Journal* 327 (2003): 316.

p. 138   *UV Foundation's goals and funders*: See www.uvfoundation.org.

p. 139   *American Academy of Dermatology*: The group's information materials for the public are available at www.aad.org/public.

p. 139   *"People shouldn't feel they can stay in the sun"*: Stephen Stone, MD, AAD president, quoted in "American Academy of Dermatology Reaffirms Position on Sun Protection Benefit of Sunscreen," news release, March 31, 2006.

p. 139   *"We don't really know whether sunscreens prevent skin cancer"*: Kathleen Fackelmann, "Melanoma Madness," *Science News*, June 6, 1998, 360.

p. 139   *"misleading and confusing"*: American Academy of Dermatology, "Tens of Millions Additional New Cases of Skin Cancer Predicted if Americans Stop Using Sunscreen," press release, March 19, 1998.

p. 140   *"numbers cruncher, not a doctor"*: Fackelmann, "Melanoma Madness."

p. 140   *The group also sent a letter to Berwick*: Letter from Roger Ceilley, immediate past president of the American Academy of Dermatology to Marianne Berwick, March 12, 1998.

p. 140   *"Research Shines Dangerous Truth on Sun Exposure"*: See American Academy of Dermatology, www.aad.org/media/background/factsheets/fact_vitamind.htm.

8. CONSUMER ACTIVISTS

p. 146   *60 Minutes segment on Alar*: "A Is for Apple," *60 Minutes*, CBS News, February 26, 1989. Quotes from Cynthia Crossen, *Tainted Truth: The Manipulation of Fact in America* (New York: Simon and Schuster, 1994), 55; Robert Bidinotto, "The Great Apple Scare," *Reader's Digest*, October 1990, 53–58.

p. 146   *Trying to quell the furor*: U.S. Food and Drug Administration, "Alar Use on

Apples," press release, March 16, 1989, www.fda.gov/bbs/topics/NEWS/
NEW00128.html.

p. 147   *"to create so many repetitions of NRDC's message":* Extracts from David
Fenton's memo were published in "How a PR Firm Executed the Alar
Scare," *Wall Street Journal,* October 3, 1989.

p. 147   *"Taking out an ad in a prestigious newspaper":* Charlotte Brody quoted in
Tina Adler, "Environmental Advantage: Marketing the Messages," *Environmental Health Perspectives* 10 (2002): A582–A585.

p. 148   *FDA analysis of:* Jean Hubinger and Don Havery, "Analysis of Consumer
Cosmetic Products for Phthalate Esters," *Journal of Cosmetic Science* 57
(2006): 127–137.

p. 148   *Several of the ads:* The various ads described here can be seen at www
.safecosmetics.org/newsroom/our_ads.cfm.

p. 148   *"make it difficult to translate the effects":* Centers for Disease Control and
Prevention, "Third National Report on Human Exposure to Environ-
mental Chemicals," July 2005, www.cdc.gov/exposurereport/report.htm.

p. 148   *CDC studies of phthalate concentrations among women:* Manori Silva et al.,
"Urinary Levels of Seven Phthalate Metabolites in the U.S. Population
from the National Health and Nutrition Examination Survey (NHANES):
1999–2000," *Environmental Health Perspectives* 112 (2004): 331–338.

p. 149   *premature breast development and sperm-related problems:* Ivelisse Colón et al.,
"Identification of Phthalate Esters in the Serum of Young Puerto Rican
Girls with Premature Breast Development," *Environmental Health Perspec-
tives* 108 (2000): 895–900; Russ Hauser et al., "DNA Damage in Human
Sperm Is Related to Urinary Levels of Phthalate Monoester and Oxidative
Metabolites," *Human Reproduction* 22 (2007): 688–695.

p. 149   *shorter AGDs:* Shanna Swan et al., "Decrease in Anogenital Distance
among Male Infants with Prenatal Phthalate Exposure," *Environmental
Health Perspectives* 113 (2005): 1056–1061.

p. 149   *"very low" phthalate exposure because they're typically washed off:* Hubinger and
Havery, "Analysis of Consumer Products for Phthalate Esters."

p. 149   *"does not have compelling evidence":* U.S. Food and Drug Administration,
Center for Food Safety and Applied Nutrition, "Phthalates and Cosmetic
Products," March 31, 2005, www.cfsan.fda.gov/~dms/cos-phth.html.

p. 149   *even when multiple cosmetic products are used:* Cosmetic Ingredient Review Expert Panel, "Dibutyl Phthalate, Diethyl Phthalate, and Dimethyl Phthalate
Re-review Summary," February 7, 2003, accessible at www.cir-safety.org/
alerts.shtml.

p. 151   *about 5 parts per billion:* Antonia Calafat et al., "Perfluorochemicals in
Pooled Serum Samples from United States Residents in 2001 and 2002,"
Environmental Science and Technology 40 (2006): 2128–2134.

p. 152   *"the right thing . . . for our environment and our health"*: Susan Hazen, acting assistant administrator of the Environmental Protection Agency's Office of Prevention, Pesticides, and Toxic Substances, "EPA Seeking PFOA Reductions," news release, January 25, 2006.

p. 152   *"does not believe there is any reason"*: U.S. Environmental Protection Agency, "Basic Information on PFOA," www.epa.gov/oppt/pfoa/pubs/pfoainfo .htm.

p. 152   *"polluting drinking water and newborn babies"*: Environmental Working Group, "EPA Fines Teflon Maker DuPont for Chemical Cover-Up," news release, December 14, 2005, www.ewg.org/node/8766.

p. 152   *when heated, Teflon can break down*: Environmental Working Group, "Canaries in the Kitchen: Teflon Toxicosis," May 14, 2003, www.ewg.org/ reports/toxicteflon.

p. 152   *On the Teflon Web site*: See www.teflon.com/Teflon/teflonissafe/index.html.

p. 153   *report about Teflon on 20/20*: "Safe or Sorry? New Evidence Reveals Dangers of Teflon," *20/20*, ABC News, transcript, November 14, 2003.

p. 156   *a chemical called Zonyl RP*: *Good Morning America*, ABC News, transcript, November 18, 2005.

p. 156   *"hid for decades that it was polluting"*: Environmental Working Group, "Former DuPont Top Expert: Company Knew, Covered Up Pollution of Americans' Blood for 18 Years," press release, November 16, 2005, www .ewg.org/node/8764.

p. 156   *the FDA informed EWG in a letter*: Letter from Laura Tarantino, director of the Office of Food Additive Safety, to Richard Wiles, December 20, 2005, www2.dupont.com/PFOA/en_US/pdf/MedAdv_FDADismissesEWG Allegations.pdf.

p. 157   *yet another story on Teflon*: *World News Tonight*, ABC News, transcript, January 25, 2006.

p. 157   *"the courage to stand up in public"*: Environmental Working Group, "EPA, DuPont Agree to Virtually Eliminate Perfluorinated Chemicals by 2015: Statement from EWG President Ken Cook," press release, January 25, 2006, www.ewg.org/node/21303.

p. 158   *"reported in a way that tries to evaluate their truth"*: Trevor Butterworth, Statistical Assessment Service, "Media Sticks Poisonous Popcorn Bags to Teflon Chemical," November 28, 2005, www.stats.org/stories/media_sticks _popcorn_teflon_nov28_05.htm.

p. 158   *"whether journalists are doing the public any favors"*: Trevor Butterworth, Statistical Assessment Service, "How Activist Groups Run the News," January 31, 2007, www.stats.org/stories/2007/how_activist_grps_jan31_2007 .htm.

p. 158   *"the scarier and more bizarre the story"*: John Stossel, *Myths, Lies, and Down-*

right Stupidity: Get Out the Shovel — Why Everything You Know Is Wrong (New York: Hyperion, 2006), 2.

p. 158   *A Michigan-based activist group:* See www.healthycar.org/about.why.php.

p. 158   *volatile organic compounds (VOCs):* Environmental Protection Agency, "Basic Information: Organic Gases (volatile organic compounds—VOCs)," www .epa.gov/iaq/voc.html.

p. 159   *relatively high VOC levels in new, parked cars:* Marion Fedoruk and Brent Kerger, "Measurement of Volatile Organic Compounds inside Automobiles," *Journal of Exposure Analysis and Environmental Epidemiology* 13 (2003): 31–41; Toshiaki Yoshida and Ichiro Matsunaga, "A Case Study on Identification of Airborne Organic Compounds and Time Courses of Their Concentrations in the Cabin of a New Car for Private Use," *Environment International* 32 (2006): 58–79.

p. 159   *"no apparent health hazard":* Jeroen Buters et al., "Toxicity of Parked Motor Vehicle Indoor Air," *Environmental Science and Technology* 41 (2007): 2622– 2629.

p. 159   *"Consumer Guide to Toxic Chemicals in Cars":* Jeff Gearhart et al., "The Consumer Guide to Toxic Chemicals in Cars: Model Year 2006/2007 Guide to New Vehicles," March 2007, www.healthycar.org/documents/ healthycarguide07.pdf.

p. 159   *exhaust fumes emitted by other vehicles:* See, for example, International Center for Technology Assessment, "In-Car Air Pollution: The Hidden Threat to Automobile Drivers," July 2000, www.icta.org/doc/In-car%20pollution %20report.pdf.

p. 159   *auto accident and other mortality statistics:* National Highway Traffic Safety Administration, "Traffic Safety Facts: 2006 Traffic Safety Annual Assessment—A Preview," July 2007, www-nrd.nhtsa.dot.gov/Pubs/810791.pdf. Figures for deaths from falls, HIV/AIDS, and gun assaults come from Arialdi Miniño et al., "Deaths: Final Data for 2004," *National Vital Statistics Reports* 55, no. 19, August 21, 2007, Centers for Disease Control and Prevention, www.cdc.gov/nchs/data/nvsr/nvsr55/nvsr55_19.pdf.

9. ANTI-AGING DOCTORS

p. 164   *"have not been evaluated or approved by A4M":* "Show Guide," Chicago Anti-Aging Exposition, Summer 2006, 1.

p. 166   *A panel of gerontology experts:* Robert Butler et al., "Biomarkers of Aging: From Primitive Organisms to Humans," *Journal of Gerontology: Biological Sciences* 59A (2004): 560–567.

p. 166   *"the equivalent of a blood pressure cuff for testing aging":* Robert Butler quoted in International Longevity Center–USA, "Growing Claims of 'Anti-Aging' Medicine Unprovable, Warns New Report from International Longevity Center–USA," news release, July 12, 2001.

p. 166   *suggested benefits of antioxidant supplements:* Alan Dangour, Victoria Sibson, and Astrid Fletcher, "Micronutrient Supplementation in Later Life: Limited Evidence for Benefit," *Journal of Gerontology: Biological Sciences* 59A (2004): 659–673.

p. 166   *"is not supported by the currently available scientific literature":* Ibid.

p. 166   *a slightly* increased *risk of dying earlier:* Goran Bjelakovic et al., "Mortality in Randomized Trials of Antioxidant Supplements for Primary and Secondary Prevention: Systematic Review and Meta-analysis," *Journal of the American Medical Association* 297 (2007): 842–857.

p. 167   *"no known dietary supplements that have been proven":* S. Jay Olshansky quoted in "'Silver Fleece' Awards Warn Consumers of Anti-Aging Misinformation," University of Illinois at Chicago, news release, February 26, 2004.

p. 167   *one popular clinic lists the following effects:* See www.ehealthspan.com.

p. 168   *GH was administered to twelve healthy older men:* Daniel Rudman et al., "Effects of Human Growth Hormone in Men over 60 Years Old," *New England Journal of Medicine* 323 (1990): 1–6.

p. 168   *"because there are so many unanswered questions":* Mary Lee Vance, "Growth Hormone for the Elderly?" *New England Journal of Medicine* 323 (1990): 52–54.

p. 168   *"the beginning of the end of aging":* Ronald Klatz, with Carol Kahn, *Grow Young with HGH* (New York: HarperCollins, 1997).

p. 168   *Subsequent research has reinforced the need for caution:* Hau Liu et al., "Systematic Review: The Safety and Efficacy of Growth Hormone in the Healthy Elderly," *Annals of Internal Medicine* 146 (2007): 104–115; Maxine Papadakis et al., "Growth Hormone Replacement in Healthy Older Men Improves Body Composition but Not Functional Ability," *Annals of Internal Medicine* 124 (1996): 708–716; Marc Blackman et al., "Growth Hormone and Sex Steroid Administration in Healthy Aged Women and Men: A Randomized Controlled Trial," *Journal of the American Medical Association* 288 (2002): 2282–2292.

p. 168   *elevated levels of IGF-1 and increased risk of cancer:* Mitchell Harman and Marc Blackman, "Use of Growth Hormone for Prevention or Treatment of Effects of Aging," *Journal of Gerontology: Biological Sciences* 59A (2004): 652–658.

p. 169   *Mice with deficiencies of growth hormone:* Ibid.

p. 169   *"libido and improved mood return within days":* See www.ehealthspan.com.

p. 170   *benefits and risks of testosterone replacement:* For a review of the research, see David Gruenewald and Alvin Matsumoto, "Testosterone Supplementation Therapy for Older Men: Potential Benefits and Risks," *Journal of the American Geriatrics Society* 51 (2003): 101–115.

p. 170   *An analysis that pooled data from 30 trials:* Rudy Haddad et al., "Testosterone and Cardiovascular Risk in Men: A Systematic Review and Meta-Analysis of Randomized Placebo-Controlled Trials," *Mayo Clinic Proceedings* 82 (2007): 29–39.

p. 170   *there are too many unknowns:* Institute of Medicine, "Testosterone and Aging: Clinical Research Directions," November 12, 2003.

p. 170   *"Until the efficacy and safety of testosterone therapy":* Dr. Dan Balzer quoted in "Testosterone Therapy Studies Should Determine Benefits First, Then Risks; Study Participants Should Be Limited, Carefully Screened," National Academies press release, November 12, 2003, www8.nationalacademies .org/onpinews/newsitem.aspx?RecordID=10852.

p. 170   *DHEA and cardiovascular death:* See, for example, Elizabeth Barrett-Connor, Kay-Tee Khaw, and Samuel Yen, "A Prospective Study of Dehydro-epiandrosterone Sulfate, Mortality, and Cardiovascular Disease," *New England Journal of Medicine* 315 (1986): 1519–1524; Elizabeth Barrett-Connor and Deborah Goodman-Gruen, "Dehydroepiandrosterone Sulfate Does Not Predict Cardiovascular Death in Postmenopausal Women: The Rancho Bernardo Study," *Circulation* 91 (1995): 1757–1760; Daksha Trivedi and Kay-Tee Khaw, "Dehydroepiandrosterone Sulfate and Mortality in Elderly Men and Women," *Journal of Clinical Endocrinology and Metabolism* 86 (2001): 4171–4177.

p. 170   *Small, short-term studies in healthy older people:* For a review, see Ketan Dhatariya and K. Sreekumaran Nair, "Dehydroepiandrosterone: Is There a Role for Replacement?" *Mayo Clinic Proceedings* 78 (2003): 1257–1273.

p. 170   *two-year randomized study:* Sreekumaran Nair et al., "DHEA in Elderly Women and DHEA or Testosterone in Elderly Men," *New England Journal of Medicine* 355 (2006): 1647–1659.

p. 171   *"DHEA is so safe":* See www.physioage.com.

p. 171   *"This issue needs to be fully addressed":* Dhatariya and Nair, "Dehydroepian-drosterone."

p. 171   *"much better form of HRT":* See www.physioage.com.

p. 172   *"the body accepts and metabolizes natural hormones":* Www.milesmd.com. Accessed September 1, 2007; no longer available.

p. 172   *little long-term research on bioidentical hormones:* Endocrine Society, "Bio-identical Hormones," Position Statement, October 2006, www.endo-society .org/publicpolicy/policy/upload/BH_Position_Statement_final_10_25_06 _w_Header.pdf.

p. 172   *An FDA analysis of 29 product samples:* Center for Drug Evaluation and Research, "Report: Limited FDA Survey of Compounded Drug Products," January 2003, www.fda.gov/CDER/pharmcomp/survey.htm.

p. 173   *"safe and has no adverse effects":* See www.infinitevitality.net.

p. 174   *medical training of Ronald Klatz and Robert Goldman:* For their official bios, see www.worldhealth.net/p/142,336.html (Klatz) and www.worldhealth .net/p/141,335.html (Goldman).

p. 174   *"break free from the medical insurance maze"*: See www.cenegenicsfoundation .org.

p. 174   *"your gateway to opportunity"*: This description was on a poster at the A4M conference I attended in Chicago, as well as in the program guide for attendees.

p. 175   *quotes from patients such as these*: Cenegenics Medical Institute, *The Complete Guide to Healthy Aging*, 2006, www.nxtbook.com/nxtbooks/wsi/patient guide/index.php.

p. 176   *science-based statement about human aging*: For an overview, see "No Truth to the Fountain of Youth," *Scientific American*, June 2002, 92–95. The full statement is available at www.quackwatch.org/01QuackeryRelatedTopics/ antiagingpp.html.

p. 177   *A4M's response to the scientific statement*: American Academy of Anti-Aging Medicine, "Official Position Statement on the Truth about Human Aging Intervention," June 2002, www.worldhealth.net/p/96,333.html.

p. 178   *"Looking at historical trends"*: Peter Schwartz, chairman of the Global Business Network, quoted in ibid. His full statement appears in *Wired* magazine, May 2002.

p. 178   *In 1900, the average life expectancy*: Centers for Disease Control and Prevention, National Center for Health Statistics, *Health, United States, 2007*, www .cdc.gov/nchs/hus.htm.

p. 178   *"Adding 80 years"*: S. Jay Olshansky and Bruce Carnes, *The Quest for Immortality: Science at the Frontiers of Aging* (New York: Norton, 2001), 87.

p. 180   *"the single most important thing an older person can do"*: John Rowe and Robert Kahn, *Successful Aging* (New York: Pantheon, 1998), 98.

p. 180   *A study of Japanese American men*: Bradley Willcox et al., "Midlife Risk Factors and Healthy Survival in Men," *Journal of the American Medical Association* 296 (2006): 2343–2350.

p. 180   *A large study of centenarians and their families*: Thomas Perls and Margery Hutter Silver, *Living to 100: Lessons in Living to Your Maximum Potential at Any Age* (New York: Basic, 1999).

p. 180   *"We'd have to wait"*: Ronald Klatz quoted in Gina Kolata, "Chasing Youth, Many Gamble on Hormones," *New York Times*, December 22, 2002.

10. GUARANTEED!

p. 183   *"walking testimonial"*: Wade Greene, "Guru of the Organic Food Cult," *New York Times* magazine, June 6, 1971, SM30.

p. 183   *"I am so healthy that I expect to live on and on"*: Carlton Jackson, *J. I. Rodale: Apostle of Nonconformity* (New York: Pyramid, 1974), 224.

p. 183   *one writer suggested that Rodale's death:* Milton Feher, "No Time for Relaxation," *New York Times,* Letters, June 27, 1971.

p. 183   *"Rodale has ruined the entire health-food industry":* Jackson, *Rodale,* 233.

p. 184   *people groped for explanations:* See, for example, Claudia Wallis, "Why Joggers Are Running Scared," *Time,* August 6, 1984, www.time.com/time/magazine/article/0,9171,921748,00.html; "Deadly Refusal," *New York Times,* August 1, 1984.

p. 184   *"often preventable":* Lynn Smaha quoted in "Cardiovascular Disease and Life Expectancy," American Heart Association, press release, December 30, 1999.

p. 184   *"Dr. Lynn Allan Smaha RIP":* This blog entry, written by Dr. Michael Eades on April 20, 2006, is available at www.proteinpower.com/drmike/2006/04/20/dr-lynn-allan-smaha-rip/.

p. 185   *men who run at least an hour a week:* Mihaela Tanasescu et al., "Exercise Type and Intensity in Relation to Coronary Heart Disease in Men," *Journal of the American Medical Association* 288 (2002): 1994–2000.

p. 186   *diet and likelihood of developing heart disease:* Frank Hu et al., "Prospective Study of Major Dietary Patterns and Risk of Coronary Heart Disease in Men," *American Journal of Clinical Nutrition* 72 (2000): 912–921.

p. 187   *"How could a person in perfect health":* William Alcott, *Vegetable Diet* (Boston: Marsh, Capen, and Lyon, 1838), 242–243.

p. 187   *those who subscribe to fatalistic beliefs:* Jeff Niederdeppe and Andrea Gurmankin Levy, "Fatalistic Beliefs about Cancer Prevention and Three Prevention Behaviors," *Cancer Epidemiology, Biomarkers and Prevention* 16 (2007): 998–1003.

p. 191   *"The more assiduously we try to guard our good health":* Arthur Barsky, *Worried Sick: Our Troubled Quest for Wellness* (Boston: Little, Brown, 1988), 158.

p. 191   *"a nation of healthy hypochondriacs":* Lewis Thomas, *The Medusa and the Snail: More Notes of a Biology Watcher* (New York: Bantam, 1980), 39.

p. 191   *"Health, like any wealth":* George Will, "Grandmother Was Right," *Newsweek,* January 16, 1989, 68.

ACKNOWLEDGMENTS

Though writing this book is something I've been thinking about for years—friends, relatives, and colleagues who have patiently listened to me ramble on about it can certainly attest to that—I could never have followed through without the contributions of a number of people.

Stan Holwitz of the University of California Press provided indispensable support, serving as chief guide, counselor, and cheerleader as I made my way through the publication process. A big thank-you goes as well to Dore Brown, Mary Renaud, and Randy Heyman for their fantastic work preparing and polishing the manuscript.

My lead research assistant, Kate McMahon, did a brilliant job gathering information, double- and triple-checking facts, and commenting on drafts. Her upbeat personality and can-do attitude made her a joy to work with. I'm also indebted to Gina Hill, Catherine Jacobs, Debra Goldschmidt, and John Gunn for their superb research support.

Ed Gamble, an award-winning editorial cartoonist for the *Florida Times-Union* in Jacksonville, kindly lent his considerable talent to the book by creating one of the illustrations. Others—including John Abramson, Linda Bacon, Phyllis Becker, Marianne Berwick, Steve Blair, Trevor Butterworth, Scottie Davis, Loren Goldfarb, Beatrice Golumb, Julie Hudtloff, Joe Miller, Jay Olshansky, Jonathan Ringel, Gary Schwitzer, Marla Shainberg, Gil Welch, and Jim Whorton—generously gave of their time by reading various chapters (in some cases, all of them) and offering thoughtful feedback and suggestions.

A special thank-you to Edward Felsenthal, my good friend for nearly 30 years and one of the most talented editors and writers I know. He advised me on this project from start to finish, sharing insights, advice, and constructive criticism that unquestionably made it a better book.

My friend Lisa Lillien, the genius behind the wildly popular Hungry Girl brand, gave me constant encouragement as well as the benefit of her tremendous creativity. And I'm deeply grateful to my sister, Emily Weaver, who always saw to it that I had much-needed diversions from my writing.

Finally, I would be remiss not to acknowledge my high school English teachers Lin Askew, James Russell, Terry Shelton, and Norman Thompson, who are among the best in the business. They have my eternal thanks for nurturing my love of language, teaching me how to write, and giving me the confidence to do it for a living. I hope this project earns a passing grade from them.

INDEX

TEXT
10/14 Janson
DISPLAY
Akzidenz Grotesk
COMPOSITOR
BookMatters, Berkeley
INDEXER
Thérèse Shere
PRINTER/BINDER
Sheridan Books, Inc.

HCOLW 612
D263

Friends of the
Houston Public Library

DAVIS, ROBERT J.
    THE HEALTHY SKEPTIC

COLLIER
11/08